Nurse Gone Strong

Published by Terri Wentzell

www.nursegonestrong.com
nursegonestrong@gmail.com

Copyright by Terri Wentzell 2017

Special Thanks:
- Book formatting and cover design by Lloyd Wentzell
- Cover photo taken by Cassie Wentzell
- Detailed editing by Ralph Filicchia and Sharon Wentzell
- My "manager" Audrey Wentzell for making sure I met my
deadlines, and my biggest cheerleader, Evelyn Wentzell - I
love you girls to the moon and back!

Nurse Gone Strong

by Terri Wentzell

Nurse Gone Strong

Table of Contents:

Preface

I cannot fully explain the joy I feel to actually have this book completed. Being a nurse myself for 20 years, I know exactly what it feels like. I understand the struggles, be they physical, emotional, relational, etc. It can be really hard for nurses to take a step back and realize that taking care of themselves is actually something that matters. We are so used to focusing on caring for others all the time, and it's easy to push our own needs to the side. I am hoping to shed some light on this issue and offer some practical solutions to a profession that so desperately needs permission to care for themselves.

I thank God from the bottom of my heart for giving me the passion and motivation to do this, and allowing me to work on this to completion. I want to thank my family for being patient with me as I have taken so much time and put so much effort into this. I could not have done this without their love and support. I hope you all enjoy this book and are truly blessed in many ways because of it. Thank you!!!

Chapter One

The Need to Care For Nurses

Nurses. They are a one-of-a-kind breed. Dedicated, hard working, caring, and sacrificing to the point of putting patients' needs above their own. If you are not a nurse yourself, chances are you know someone in your family or circle of friends who is. They most often take on that role in their family lives, and maybe even in their circle of friends, as well as on the job. It is in their nature to be caretakers. So what do we know about caretakers? They are usually the ones forever caring for the needs of others, yet never worrying about caring for themselves. They give, give, and give some more, always being sure others' needs are met before worrying about themselves. We've all seen it.

And this can be true of mothers caring for their children, people caring for aging parents, and other similar situations. But for nurses especially, working in the conditions they frequently do with long hours, minimal breaks, excessive stress, and overloaded patient assignments, this issue is very serious. When a nurse has no time, ability, or tools to help him or her actually care for themselves, this can lead to job burnout, higher risk for injury on the job, poor health, poor job satisfaction and much more. I believe, as a nurse myself for 20 years, it is time to take care of our nurses. They are the backbone of healthcare, usually the ones patients most trust and remember during hospitalizations, and they deserve better!

> "Nurses are a unique kind. They have this insatiable need to care for others, which is both their greatest strength and fatal flaw."
> -Dr. Jean Watson

These are the reasons I am writing this book. I see it every day, and I've heard my share of horror stories to know it is everywhere. I want to be a voice for nurses to take a stand for their own health and well-being. It matters! Some may say that nurses should be healthy to be a good example to their patients. While this may or may not be true, it is not the focus of this book. That's not the point here. It's not my position to put some other demands on nurses to better fulfill their role. Nurses are told enough things to do every day, and the last thing someone wants to be "told" is to be healthy. The work environment alone can be very detrimental to a nurse's well-being, and this will be further addressed later on. It goes beyond just trying to be healthy.

Managers or nursing directors may say that nurses should take better care of themselves to improve work performance and decrease sick days taken. Again, not my point. This is not something you force on anyone, let alone nurses. Nurses are people, and all people need to be inspired and empowered to live a life of health for their OWN benefit; not to benefit someone else.

My point for this book is to spread awareness and motivation to nurses everywhere to take some time in caring for themselves. I want them to realize their full value, and how taking time to care for themselves can improve their overall life satisfaction, let alone the benefits on the job. Take pride in yourself, your health, your role in society and just plain enjoy life more! Why not? You deserve that, and then some. Let's do this.

Why do people become nurses? You have to have a desire to help others first, and I believe that is what drives most nurses to go into this field. Maybe your mom was a nurse, or someone else in the family, and this encouraged you to look into this field (my mom was a nurse, and this is what prompted me to look into nursing for myself). Maybe you or a loved one was a former patient who had an amazing experience with nurses who cared for you, and you wanted to give back. Some people enter the nursing career because they hate the thought of a 9-5 Monday through Friday work week (another plus for me!). Nursing can be extremely flexible with many scheduling options that can fit almost any need. This works well for moms with young kids, or others who just want more flexibility in their work week.

A nursing degree can take you far in life. There are so many avenues one can take with this career, and one job can be completely different from the next. The possibilities are truly endless. And let's not ignore the obvious... nursing pays well! Although It's important to point out, we have all had shifts that leave you feeling like NO amount of money could actually put an accurate value on what you just went through. However, nurses pay in general is clearly a bonus that weighs heavily on people's decisions to enter this field. But money aside, nursing is NOT for everyone.

What does it take to be a nurse? Sure, you need a desire to help others, but it goes way beyond that. We all know very nice people who would give you the shirt off their back, but they would rather have any other profession on earth before being a nurse. For some, it's the blood, bodily fluids, horrendous wounds, bed pans, and other not so pleasant aspects of the job that turn people completely off from wanting anything to do with this job. Do all nursing jobs deal with this stuff? Not necessarily, however, you do need to make it through nursing school first - and you are sure to get your fill of grossness there. You can have a desire to help people all you want, but if you have a weak stomach, this may not be the profession for you. It takes a special kind of person to get past all that. Ask any nurse who has been in the profession for a while - you pretty much can't gross them out. They've seen it all!

Let's take a look at a day in the life of a nurse and why this book is so crucial. If you have been a nurse for any amount of time, chances are you have known what it is like to work 12 or even 16 hour shifts with minimal breaks to feed yourself, go to the bathroom, or even take a moment to decompress. You run on empty for hours, and this can be empty of food, water, and emotional strength.... but you keep going. Your coworkers need you. Your patients need you. The acuity of your patients demands this.

You spread yourself so thin in every direction, leaving little strength left to barely give report at the end of your shift. You may need to change assignments on a minute's notice, and be expected to have everything in order for handoffs. You may be required to make split second decisions that could determine life or death for a patient, all while keeping track of the 800 other things on the "to-do" list in your head. You are emotionally available to not only your patients, but your patients' family members (and sometimes this task is even more demanding!). You can be all-out drained after a long code on your patient, only to have them expire... then go take report on the next patient without letting it faze you.

Then let's not forget the workplace stressors of dealing with budget cuts and staffing issues. Feeling frustrated with less, when, at times, you really could use a lot more to get your job done effectively and in the safest way for your patients.

The physical demands on nurses? The list goes on and on. Where do we begin? Long shifts can be filled with lots of bending, stretching, reaching, heavy lifting, pushing and carrying equipment, miles of walking, and much more. Back injuries are a major issue with nursing because of the huge physical demands that are part of the job. Yes, efforts have been made to decrease this issue with the development of lifting equipment for patients, and that has proven to be helpful. However, there are always the unexpected times of a patient falling during a transfer, a walk, or slipping out of a bed or chair when the hero nurse comes to the rescue to catch the patient. There is no lift equipment in emergency situations like this. The nurse dives in to save the day, and the potential for injury is great.

Then there are the times when you are lifting heavy equipment, whether that be IV pumps, monitors, oxygen tanks, heavy dialysis bags, etc... and there are no lifting machines to do this type of stuff for you. Some of that stuff is seriously heavy! Nurses have the potential of slipping on wet floors just after housekeeping mops the patient's room, or from spills of bodily fluids causing a hazardous situation. Tripping over equipment, cables, or IV lines, or even being injured from dropped tools or heavy equipment are all possibilities for physical injury.

And last but not least, nurses are physically abused. Somewhere along the line in your nursing career, I'm sure you remember (or will encounter, if you are a new nurse) being punched, grabbed, pulled, scratched, kicked, pushed, or had something thrown at you by a patient. I know I can recall a few of these instances myself. Not to mention, this can include verbal abuse as well. And this could be from a patient, a coworker, or even a physician who thinks he or she has more power than God himself, feeling the need to belittle a nurse for whatever reason. But the nurse must take it all in stride, continue on with his or her tasks, and give their best care... regardless of how they feel.

Nurses are exposed to infectious diseases, medications that can be toxic if handled incorrectly, and could be exposed to excess radiation depending on where they work. Needle sticks can and do occur, subjecting nurses to the risks of acquiring such diseases as HIV and hepatitis B or C. Safety measures are always in place for this type of thing, but accidents do happen, and there are no guarantees.

Is it really any wonder that nursing ranks up near the top for one of the most dangerous jobs out there? Wow. Now I know that not every shift of every nursing job involves all of that which I just discussed, and by no means am I trying to scare off anyone from thinking of becoming a nurse. But those situations and circumstances are very real possibilities and realities of many nurses' lives every day. It takes a lot out of someone, physically and emotionally, to deal with that type of job.

You can also see how a nurse may not feel like they have anything left to give after a shift to actually pay any attention to their own needs. That seems to fall to the wayside far more often that it should. But who is looking after the nurse? Who speaks up on their behalf for their health and well-being? Who gives them permission, encouragement, motivation and support in this area so the nurses themselves actually feel cared for and well? Not enough

> "Self-compassion is simply giving the same kindness to ourselves that we would give to others."
> -Christopher Germer

people, that's for sure. Again, that is my motivation for writing this book.

Let's take a moment to think of some "what-ifs". What if nurses actually felt good coming and going from work most days? What if nurses could decrease their stress levels significantly without having to change their job? What if nurses had better sleep and felt more refreshed every day? What if nurses felt physically strong making all those heavy tasks a lot easier to perform while also decreasing their risk of injury? What if nurses could get rid of that afternoon (or 3 am) crash of feeling like they need yet another cup of coffee just to make it through the next hour? What if nurses had a new increasing energy that made a world of difference in getting through a shift? What if nurses felt mentally and emotionally well, making it easier for them to cope with difficult situations on the job? What if nurses became the envy of all other professions because they took such excellent care of themselves that everyone else wished they could have that same kind of health, happiness, strength, physique, energy, balance and overall wellness that nurses posses? Ha-ha! Now that would be awesome. I always say, you have to dream big, or don't bother.

We all know that some circumstances are beyond our control in certain aspects of the job. Not everything can always be made better when emergencies come into play in this type of environment, and bad days are still going to happen. But I am absolutely certain that things can (and should) be better than they are. In a perfect world, all people in all types of jobs would have low stress, plenty of breaks, low risk for injury, decent hours, feel appreciated, and have positive emotional experiences every day – thus causing zero harm to their own health and wellness. This is a tough combination to find in any job, for sure, let alone nursing. However, it doesn't have to seem so far out of reach to the point where it's not even worth bothering to do anything about it. Nurses put up with a lot more on any given day than many people of other professions would ever dare dream. They need to be taken care of. They need to know that their health and well-being matter. They need to know that they can be and feel strong. They need to be encouraged to take care of themselves for the sake of their own happiness and fulfillment in life.

Nurses are strong people in many ways, but they need to be strong for themselves in the long run. What good is it to be so sacrificial in the desire to care for your patients when you take such a beating on yourself to the point that you are then no good to anyone? It's all good to go the extra mile sometimes, but please don't forget that you matter too. I've been there.

I know the guilt you can feel when you are being told to go to lunch when you're patient has a million things going on, and some other nurse with a busy assignment of her own is supposed to cover for you. It feels wrong. So you either refuse to go, or you inhale your food so quickly that you nearly choke, all in the name of your patient's safety and your coworker's sanity.

Other times you may try getting by on the candy or other junk sitting at the nurses' station that some family members or co-workers brought in, hoping that will sustain you until your shift is over. And let's face it, that stuff shows up all the time, and it is most often something that is NOT good for you! It can be hard to resist when you don't have time for a real lunch break, or you're just too tired and stressed to care what you're shoving in your mouth. Some days you might be 9 hours into your shift by the time you realized you haven't even had one sip of water all day.

Or maybe you ran around so much on your 12 hour shift that the thought of any organized exercise for yourself during the week is thrown out the window. You're exhausted, and moving more might be the last thing you want to think about.

You might agree to stay extra hours because the unit is so short staffed, even when you are already overtired and you have to be back early the next morning (or evening). Nurses can feel pressure to show up for work when they're sick so they won't make more work for their colleagues. Your own need of sleep and rejuvenation is cut short for the good of the unit and your patients, putting your needs on the back burner once again.

Sometimes the stress of a bad shift can cause nurses to go into the "screw-it-all" mode, meaning that they will binge eat (or drink) on whatever comfort food (or alcoholic beverage) of choice may be tempting them at the time. This may be harmless every once in a while, but this can also become a detrimental habit to a lot of nurses if done too much, thus furthering down that spiral of poor health for the nurse. This needs to be helped. Nurses need to be taken care of, most importantly, by themselves. No one else is going to do it for them.

Chapter Two

What Can Be Done?

So what do we do about all of this? Can anything be done? Is this too huge of a task to approach? My answer is no. With all the obstacles we just spoke about, it may seem like an enormous mess to try and fix, but I truly believe that there are things we can do to help the well-being of nurses everywhere. Can we fix every problem that exists in the nursing career? No, but improvements can be made, and we can become more aware of how issues come up. We need to break things down into different areas, and attack problems one by one. This is what the following chapters will get into in further detail.

For now, I want nurses to first realize their value. This is a must. When you don't even value yourself, you are not going to bother caring for yourself. Think of all the ways you are of value in your life; not just your job alone. What are you responsible for? Who depends on you? In what ways have you added value to the lives of others? What accomplishments are you proud of? Focus on these things and praise yourself for a job well done. This is so important! Love yourself first, then caring for yourself will be something that's important to you instead of the dead last thing you think about every day.

Now I'm going to put a spin on this that you may not have thought of. Yes, let's care of the poor nurse who is so giving and always puts other's needs first. But I ask you this - are you possibly playing the role of the martyr? Sometimes it's easy to play the victim with our lifestyle of always caring for others. Do you know what being a martyr does? It provides a convenient distraction for you to not look at what disciplines and goals you are ignoring in your own life. How can you possibly be expected to go to the gym when you have to care for everyone all the time? You don't need to address your own vulnerabilities or shortcomings when you're always focused on taking care of everyone else. It's actually easier this way. You don't need to take personal responsibility. Just project the blame outward because you have so much to do in taking care of everything else.

Martyrs sometimes truly don't know how to love themselves very well. They find value in caring for others to the point of if they stop doing that, they may feel completely useless. They don't know how to validate themselves. Martyrs think they are the only ones that can do it "right", so they have to be the ones to do it all the time. They have to be the care taker. After all, it might hurt your ego to think that sometimes people can actually get along without you doing everything for them all the time. You may be seeking praise as a reward for all you're doing. You want to be validated. But it will never be enough, and you keep going and going on this road, all the while conveniently ignoring any and all things in your own life that need to be addressed. Let's fix this right now, and take a moment to think of your motives. Does this fit you? Stop right there if it does, and face it. Step back for a moment and look at your own life and what you may be ignoring right in front of your own nose. Are you running from caring for yourself? Are you using your lifestyle or career as a scapegoat for not addressing your own issues? Think about it.

What are your dreams? Your goals? What are you striving for? What defines you? Take a moment and think about those things. It all matters in the big scheme of taking care of yourself. First realize that you are only limited by the walls you build yourself. Why can't you have more? Why don't you deserve more? You are the only one holding yourself back from anything better. Don't settle for some mediocre life trying to barely skate by with your health. If you don't go after what you want, you'll never have it.

Have you ever thought of your body as a gift? Well it's the only one you get during this life here on earth, so why not treat it with the utmost respect it deserves?

After all, it's the only place you have to live! If someone were to give you a treasured gift that was supposed to last your whole lifetime and it served you well in a million different ways, would you choose to treat it poorly? Hopefully not, yet this is what so many of us do on a daily basis with our own bodies. Your body is a gift from God; and amazing machine that is completely mind blowing to think of all its intricate details. Treasure that! Empower that machine to function at its best!

Now take a second and think of your patients. How many horrible situations have you seen? How many heart breaking stories and gut wrenching situations have you winced at? How much sadness have you witnessed in your time as a nurse? The stories are endless for many of us. Now I want you to think of how many of those situations could have possibly been prevented with certain lifestyle behaviors. Many.

> "The first wealth is health."
> -Ralph Waldo Emerson

It astounds me to realize how many diseases are completely preventable with the right lifestyle behaviors. How much heartache could have been saved? How many more years could have been enjoyed? How much higher quality of life could have been attained? Why is it that as nurses we see this stuff every day, we know all the risks and the outcomes, we see all the devastation, yet we don't make the necessary changes in our own life to prevent these very tragedies? Now I am not judging nor blaming nurses alone here. Poor health habits are a personal choice - regardless of profession. I know there are smokers out there who know very well all the risks of smoking, yet they still do it. There are people who know very well that fast food isn't good for them, yet they make their daily drive-thru run at McDonald's. We all know exercise is beneficial, yet so many of us wouldn't dare start... we're too busy. You have to decide. You have to want better. Nurses, start caring. This is your life, your future, and your dreams all at stake. Don't settle for less!!!

> **"Treatment without prevention is simply unsustainable."**
> **-Bill Gates**

I don't know about you, but I would much rather rely on prevention than treatment. Being treated for any disease is not fun. It is often very costly, time consuming, uncomfortable, life disrupting, and depressing. Nurses see this every day. Who wants to be in and out of hospitals, possibly needing major operations, taking multiple different medications a day, and needing someone else to care for you all the time rather than being able to care for yourself? Not me. Healthcare these days isn't healthcare... it's "sick care". They take care of the sick. I'd much rather focus on being healthy, so I don't need to rely on "sick care". Each and every one of us has the power in our own hands to do this. No exceptions.

Think of your car for a moment. Do you take it for routine oil changes and make sure your fluids are all in check? How about checking your tire pressure? Rotating your tires? What is all that? Maintenance. You do these things to make sure your car is running well and functioning properly. So why don't we do the necessary preventative maintenance with our own physical bodies? So often we treat our bodies as we want, then pay the big price to fix everything later.

> "Discipline is the bridge between goals and accomplishment."
> -Jim Rohn

That would be like never bothering to get an oil change on your car and just pay for a new engine once it seized. Or don't worry about ever rotating your tires because you'll just buy a whole new set a lot sooner than you would have needed to if you had done the proper maintenance. Doesn't make a whole lot of sense. One difference with a car - you can buy a new one if it's really that bad, but you only get one body.

Excuses are a dime a dozen, and everyone has some. Lose 'em. Excuses aren't your friend, they are what holds you back from getting what you want and enjoying life. Time to rethink what you really want, and realize that you have full power to control the future of your health and well-being. No one else can do that for you. At the very least, if you are not interested in losing your excuses, then realize and admit where your future might be headed. You need to take full responsibility for that.

So how do we start this? First, you have to decide. Decide that you want this. Decide that you are not interested in a life of illness and less quality than you deserve. Decide that you are worth more than what you have previously believed. Decide that you will make the changes necessary to help yourself feel better in every way. That is where you begin. If you can't make it to that point yet, then you are not ready for the rest of this book. Good intentions mean nothing. Deciding to do something and sticking to it, is everything. You can do that, but no one else can do it for you. It needs to be real, it needs to be sincere, and it needs to come from your heart. Be true to yourself, be honest, and do this with all the strength you have within you. Ignore the little voice trying to tell you that you can't do it. YES YOU CAN.

Eight Tips for Creating New Habits

1. Commit to 30 days - This is all the time it takes to typically make a new habit automatic.

2. Make it daily - Consistency is key when trying to start a new habit. You'll have better luck with an everyday plan rather than every few days.

3. Start simple - Don't try to change everything at once! It is not realistic to do a major life overhaul in 30 days. Start small and work your way up.

4. Remind yourself - Place reminders around your house to help you execute your goals.

5. Stay consistent - Try doing something at the same time and same place every day. It's easier to stick to something with familiar cues.

6. Get a buddy - There is strength in numbers! Have a buddy to help keep you motivated when you feel like quitting.

7. Replace lost needs - If you are giving up something, make sure you are replacing needs you've lost with something positive.

8. Allow for failure - You will make mistakes... don't worry! Not everything is successful immediately. Just keep going.

Chapter Three

One Size Doesn't Fit All

When it comes to all things health and fitness, the information overload out there can really blow your mind. I get that. We hear study after study proving one theory, and for as many of those you find proving that point, there are just as many studies proving the exact opposite. Now I understand a lot of that has to do with how the studies were run, and how accurate they really were, but the average person out there has no idea how to decipher that information on their own to get a true answer. All we hear on the news is "studies have shown"... so then we believe whatever follows. Or the other situation that we see is people believing things for YEARS based on a few studies done in the past, yet now the "new" studies prove that it was all wrong and the exact opposite is true. This makes me insane. Studies can be extremely helpful and are a very important tool, don't get me wrong... but I think it's easy to see where people get confused with findings that are reported and they have no idea what to believe.

A great example of this is the nutritionist from back in the 1950's named Ancel Keys. He did a study on several countries (it started out to include 22, yet he only reported findings from 7) to prove the correlation between saturated fat and heart disease. Keys, however, committed a major violation of scientific research. He was guilty of selection bias. He only used the data that supported his hypothesis, and tossed the data that did not fit with what he was trying to prove. He shaped the data to support his theory. He then took this information and spread it far and wide.

Before you know it, doctors everywhere were telling patients to cut out all saturated fat. Everyone was advised to eat a low-fat, high-carbohydrate diet that was "heart healthy". However, when later researchers analyzed his data using ALL original countries and all collected data, the link between saturated fat causing high cholesterol and heart disease was not found.

It is now more widely believed that sugar is actually more of the culprit in causing heart disease, along with so many other chronic diseases. But for years and years, after being told by doctors, commercials and every magazine you picked up that we need to eat low fat diets to prevent heart disease, we have only seen people continue to get fatter and sicker. This is such a good example of the public just going along with a "study" that they thought they could trust.

I am not writing all this to make us all skeptics of every study we hear about from now on, but simply for this reason - to help you take it all with a grain of salt. We hear about medical studies all the time as nurses. As I said before, studies are great, I definitely reference them from time to time, and they can be extremely helpful. Just don't put all your eggs in one basket when it comes to your own health. Read a lot. Read people's responses and criticisms to studies. Read related books on the topic of certain studies. But most importantly, be your OWN study. What do I mean by that? It's huge, and probably the single most important topic I will write about in this book.

Diet

We are all extremely different human beings. Am I right? That is one of the most mind blowing concepts for me to wrap my head around when you truly think of how many people are in this world, and there are no two exactly alike. Crazy. Just look at the difference from one nurse to the next. Nurses are all taught basically the same stuff in school, yet their own individual nursing style certainly comes out at the bedside. But it's a great thing! After all, that's what makes the world work, right? Not only do we have different interests, likes and dislikes, we are chemically not all the same either. Our bodies are different in SO many ways. This is why (as nurses we see this all the time) certain medications have one effect on one person, and another effect on someone else. Medicine isn't black and white because no two humans are the same. We can guess what is most likely to be helpful, but until you see how someone responds to a certain medication or certain treatment, you can never be ABSOLUTELY sure.

And if this is true, then shouldn't we treat our bodies the same way when it comes to health and fitness? I say yes. You may have heard of the term "bio-individuality" thrown around in certain places recently. What this term is eluding to is that no one diet works for everyone. We are all different with different genetic make-ups, therefore we each have our own individual needs. General diet guidelines may not always work for everyone. This is what I mean when I say "be your own study". Be a detective when it comes to your own body's response to how certain foods affect you.

We've all seen the pencil thin people who are out there eating whatever they want whenever they want. Right? And then the others complaining that if they eat a single bite of a bagel, it's an automatic inch onto their waist line. While I do think there is help for both of those groups of people (let's face it, being pencil thin and eating junk doesn't mean you're healthy), the fact is obvious that different people respond differently to the same eating habits, or same types of food.

Some people get abdominal pains and brain fog with wheat in their diet. Other's seem to have no problem in that area at all. Some can't tolerate dairy, others seem just fine with it. Some don't do well with nightshade vegetables, and others tolerate them very well. Some thrive on a vegetarian diet, while others feel horrible and weak without some animal protein. Be your own study. Find out what type of eating is most in sync with your own unique physiology.

This is why when asked by clients in the past to "just tell me what to eat", my answer is usually no. First, this takes all the thinking out of your own head so you can run on autopilot. This is never good in the long run. Second, I don't know how certain foods are going to affect you, only you do. We can talk about options and ideas, but I will rarely ever write out meal by meal, day by day eating plans for someone else to blindly follow. This can be a helpful way to start out for some, but is not always helpful in the long run.

When we let others make decisions and reason for us, we are choosing to stay oblivious. We choose to remain in that helpless state of requiring someone else to tell us what to do. In this submission to someone else's authority, we essentially give all our own power away, and take all the responsibility off ourselves. This will never help you down the road. It may help in the short term for you to maybe lose a few pounds, but for the long haul you will be left with no ability of your own to make decisions that will be right for you... because you won't know how. You've trained yourself into thinking you need someone else to tell you what to do. In a sense, this makes us very lazy, and it gives us the permission to put the blame on someone else.

It's your life, your body, your health. Learn to listen to what your body is telling you, so you can learn how to care for it for the long haul. Don't play the victim here. It's your job, your responsibility, and you can do it.

However, there is one common thread for total health when it comes to eating that HAS to go across the board, no matter what type of diet seems best for you. There is NO diet out there where anyone is thriving on processed food. None. If you want the best health for yourself, your number one goal is reducing (or eliminating all together) your intake of processed food. Fresh is always better, no matter what. This is non-negotiable across the board.

Workouts

If we're all different people with different likes and dislikes, then it only makes sense that people are going to gravitate towards physical activity that they enjoy and steer clear of the ones that they don't like so much, right? And for whatever activities that person enjoys, the next person down the line could completely despise that type of exercise and actually find enjoyment in the very thing you hate doing. All exercises are not for all people. Yup, once again, we're all different, and that's okay. I personally hate running long distances. I would rather scrub my kitchen floor on my hands and knees for hours than train for a marathon. For me, it's boring, monotonous, and I just want it to end. And I'm sure there are some people reading this right now who LOVE running, and good for you! This is where it's not worth arguing with people about how they should be doing YOUR workout and not the activity they keep going back to because they enjoy it.

> **"The secret to getting ahead is getting started."**
> **-Mark Twain**

But I will say one thing about running - you should at least make sure you know how to run if and when you may need to in life! Whether you train for long endurance runs, 5K's or you like sprints, you should be able to run in some capacity in the event you ever NEED to rely on running to save your life. You may need to run from an attacker at some point, save your child from something dangerous, or just run away from a dangerous situation. Don't make it such a foreign activity that you are not able to do it if and when it may be needed!

Whatever type of routine motivates you, keeps you active, is effective for you, and keeps you coming back for more is most likely a good fit for your interests and needs. It does no good for someone to force you into a kickboxing class if you absolutely hate it. That's not going to motivate you to come back again.

So first we choose things we think we may enjoy. Next, see what kind of results you get with that type of program. If you think it's fun, yet you're not able to meet any of your fitness goals you were hoping to reach, then it may be time to tweak something a bit. Some people have great results with one type of exercise routine, and others may not get such speedy results. It's okay sometimes to say "that's not really a fit for me"... you just learned how to listen to your body! Good for you. I tell people all the time to be their own personal trainer, in a sense. You know your body best and you know how certain exercises feel on your body better than anyone else. A trainer telling you to do "10 more" when you have a sharp pain somewhere, needs to be told about that pain. You know what it feels like - they don't unless you tell them. Trainers can be great for showing you how to push past your limits in your head, but it also can be a fine line between pushing forward, and pushing too much. Learn to recognize that and use that skill to know the difference.

Intuitive training is a remarkable solution here. This means that you basically listen and take cues from your own body when it comes to your workouts. This is pretty much how I train myself, and I find it very effective and enjoyable! Intuitive training involves being in tune with what exercises may be right for you at the time, how hard you should be pushing, and how much rest you may need in between exercises. I very rarely follow a strict workout program for myself. I plan it on my own from day to day based on how I feel, how much energy is in my tank, what aches or pains I may have, and what I feel may need the most work.

This may sound completely disorganized to some, but I find it very helpful. If I AM following some sort of program, I will often adjust where I need to depending on my body's needs, and I find that extremely helpful. For someone totally new to this idea, you may need some guidance from a trainer or someone familiar with this to get you going. With some direction and general ideas, you can learn to do this. Once you get to know how your body responds, you will have a better grasp of seeing how this works.

We all have those days when we just aren't feeling it. We're trying hard, thought we were going to have an awesome workout, but it's just not happening today. As frustrating as that may feel, just let it be. First be proud of yourself that you showed up and tried. And second, you recognized that it's just not going well today. Your body may be telling you something... like "I just don't have it in me today". I have learned over the years to completely embrace this, and let it be. It's okay. Not only is that liberating, but it's the right thing to do. If a trainer or class instructor is telling you to push it to the max, or lift heavier when you're body is NOT cooperating, that's when injuries can occur if we aren't in tune with what our body is trying to tell us. Listen to it.

> "If you listen to your body when it whispers, you will never have to listen to it scream."
> -unknown

Let go of the guilt of not going as heavy or as hard as you wanted to. Let go of feeling like you're going to disappoint your trainer. Let go of the competition going on in your head with the person next to you in the gym. Let it go. You will be better off for it in the long run, and will avoid many injuries this way. When our bodies are tired and we're trying to push them past a point that feels okay, that's when we get sloppy with form and injuries are far more likely to occur. I have learned this the hard way many times. I am still a work in progress (with everything in my life!), but I am getting better at letting this go and surrendering when my body is telling me "enough". And that goes for maybe passing on certain exercises all together sometimes. If your legs are super sore from a workout you did a day or two ago, and your trainer or instructor wants you to do heavy squats that day, maybe that's not such a great idea. Speak up! You know best, regardless of their agenda for your workout for that day.

On the other hand, you will have days that you are crushing your workout, and when it's done... you're not! On days you have more to give, then by all means, give more! Sometimes you don't know where that extra energy showed up from or why it's there, but take advantage of it. Those are the days to do extra reps, or go another mile, or add on an extra workout on top of what you just did. Listen to what your body is saying, and when it says "I'm not done yet, I've got more to give", take advantage of that! That's a beautiful thing. Don't waste it. In all your workouts, tweak things as needed, and watch and listen for how your body responds. This is the most crucial step in taking the very best care of yourself.

Awareness

Do you ever really pay attention to what you're doing, feeling, thinking, experiencing on a daily basis? How many of you have driven to work, pulled into your parking space, and then realized you have no idea how you go there? You have no remembrance of driving for all that time? I have for sure. Have you ever sat down in front of the television with a bag of some snack food and finished the entire thing without really tasting and experiencing any of it and wonder how it disappeared so fast? How can this happen? This is the all too common problem of lacking awareness. Not being present in the moments that are happening around us. We let our minds run on auto pilot so often, not being engaged in the present moment at all. This is a dangerous trap. This is where we get into trouble! It's when we look back on our day at the end of it all and say "how did I let all that happen?" or "why didn't I do x,y or z today like I wanted to?" We can have a more clear and understood path for our day ahead of us, our intentions and our reactions to things, if we start practicing some awareness (or mindfulness as we could call it). When we take control back from our aimlessly wandering thoughts, good things can happen! You actually own what you are doing rather than just letting it all happen around you.

So how do we do this? I think a great place to start is just with your breathing. We breathe automatically every moment of our lives, but do we ever really think about it? Take a second to just sit still (or before you even get out of bed in the morning) and just be aware of your breath. Notice the flow of the air going in and out. Notice your chest rising and falling. Picture the air filling your lungs each time. Don't make any effort to change anything about how you are breathing, rather just notice it happening.

If you like, then you can notice it in stages. Pay attention to the air first filling your abdomen. You may actually push the belly out and use your diaphragm to allow your belly to swell. Next, raise your ribs through dilating the thoracic cage. This fills the middle section of the lungs. Expand the lungs without straining. Lastly, allow the lungs to completely fill by raising the collar bones and filling up to the very top. Think of this sequence as pouring a glass of water. The bottom fills first, then middle, then top. When you are ready to exhale, go backwards in that same order. Empty the top, then middle, and then push all remaining air out of the bottom. Notice how it is all gently released. This is being present in the moment. You are totally aware of what is going on with your breathing... something that we don't pay attention to 99% of the time, yet it happens constantly. This is mindfulness.

Mindfulness is a brain training practice that can interrupt the unconscious random happenings that we

> **"One should become master of one's mind rather than let one's mind master him."**
> **-Nichiren Daishonin**

often find filling our lives on any given day. It switches our brain activity to the prefrontal cortex. This is the part of the brain that is responsible for planning and carrying out activities necessary to reach goals. It regulates impulse control and emotional reactions, and also plays a role in helping us ignore external distractions. We need this!!! Become friends with your prefrontal cortex.

Meditation is practiced by remaining present and satisfied in the moment. This transcends thought process. One can become aware that they are not their thoughts, but that there is an awareness that exists independent of thought. This begins with concentration. Then thought activity starts to decrease, and a focused awareness becomes more spontaneous. Meditation works best when done every day, and preferably at the same time each day. Be sure you are in a quiet and peaceful atmosphere, and sit with your spine straight and vertical. Relaxation is also a byproduct of meditation. So we become more aware, and also more relaxed. There are many apps you can download right on your phone that can help guide you in meditation, breathing and relaxation. They will even give you reminders if you've gone too long without taking a step back to breathe! This is a great tool if you need reminders for this kind of activity.

The beautiful thing that happens when we start to become more aware is that we realize things don't have to be as out of control as we make them. It's a relief! This can start the process of being aware of all kinds of things that can help with your journey in all things health and fitness. Be aware of how you feel when you eat certain foods. Be aware of when you're actually satisfied and don't need to continue eating. Be aware of how you feel when you do or don't get exercise on any given day. Be aware of what exercises feel good and what ones do not. What do you like about the ones you enjoy? What is it that you don't like about the exercises you don't enjoy? Make mental notes of all of these findings. You may learn an awful lot about yourself that you never realized!

Journaling can be very helpful here. If you have never tried this, I would recommend giving it a chance. I admit, I do not journal all the time and it is not a regular activity of mine. However, I have definitely used this practice at certain times in my life and I find it very effective for truly understanding my own thoughts, intentions, future goals, and where I may have gone wrong at times.

Whether it's journaling your food intake, your feelings on certain foods, your workouts, or just your thoughts on your entire journey of health and fitness, this can be a huge eye opener. It's one thing to mindlessly snack on food all day without realizing it, and it's a whole new ballgame when you have to write it all down. You may think twice about grabbing a second cookie when you know you have to write that down... even if you're the only one who sees it. Journaling has power. Sometimes it doesn't take long to see where you may need some adjustments after reading what you've been journaling. Journaling helps keep you accountable for what is truly going on.

For some, this becomes a daily habit and almost necessary to keep their thoughts in line. That's great if that's what it turns out to be for you. If it's just a temporary tool to help you learn something more about yourself that in turn helps you create better habits, then I'm all for that as well. Bottom line, it's worth a try if you've never done it.

When you truly begin to grasp the concept of awareness and really start to understand how unique your own body is from everyone else's, this is where the journey really takes off. Now you start actually listening to your body instead of fighting it. You surrender to the fact that your body knows best... not some strict diet routine or insane workout program that you hate doing in the name of fitness. And maybe, just maybe, you start treating yourself with a little more kindness. This, above all, is the greatest gift you can give yourself.

Chapter Four

Food First

> **"Let food be thy medicine, and medicine be thy food."**
> **-Hippocrates**

Yes, food first. Food is your number one defense against disease and poor health. Notice I did not say medicine, vitamin pills, or supplements. Sure, there may be a need for medications of some sort in your lifetime, and you may want to experiment with some healthy supplements somewhere along the line, but you are wasting your time relying on pills if you are not first EATING your medicine in the form of food. Get it from the real source first... not some manmade pill created in a factory somewhere.

It makes me laugh to see some people eating junk all day long, yet spending half of their weekly paycheck on expensive supplements that are going to keep them "young and healthy" forever. They are negating every possible benefit of those supplements with eating a crappy diet. Not to mention, many nutrients cannot be properly absorbed without specific enzymes that are only present in the whole foods they originally come from. You may be wasting your time and money buying these special pills if they are not even able to be absorbed in that isolated supplement form, minus the necessary enzymes for the job. Food for thought. Save your money, and start by eating right first.

There is no greater act of self care than to carefully select and prepare healthy, fresh food to nourish your body every day. The food you eat will have the greatest impact on your overall fitness and energy levels as well. Most people have no idea how good their body was truly designed to feel until they do a full overhaul on their food choices, realizing how much better life can feel when you eat the way our bodies function best. This is an enormous topic and we will not cover everything there possibly is to talk about in this chapter, but I will try to hit the basics.

Processed Food

Let's start with processed food. So many of us (especially busy nurses who work long hours) rely on pre-packaged processed foods that have a shelf life that could out-live their own life. Processed foods are filled with additives, preservatives, and other potentially harmful ingredients that are only hurting you in the long run. The scary part is that so many of these ingredients are actually banned in other countries because of their potential harm to humans. That is crazy. Don't let yourself be part of this experiment.

Apple Crunch Bowl

-one small organic apple, chopped

-2 Tablespoons unsweetened coconut flakes

-2 Tablespoons nuts (I like almond slivers and crushed walnuts)

-small handful of dried cranberries

-1/2- 3/4 cup plain kefir

-dash of cinnamon

Add apple, coconut flakes, nuts and cranberries to a bowl; pour kefir over and top with a dash of cinnamon. If desired, lightly toast nuts and coconut flakes in a toaster oven first to give a slight golden brown look and deeper taste.

Have you ever tried to pronounce all the ingredients that are in some packaged food you have bought? It's tough, isn't it? The problem with processed, packaged food is that so much of what's in it, is not food. Butylated hydroxyanisole and butylated hydrozyttoluene are not easy to say, nor do they sound like any ingredients my grandma used to use with her homemade recipes. That's because they are preservatives that can affect your neurologic system, possibly alter behavior, and potentially cause cancer. Yet these ingredients are in so many packaged foods right on the shelf of your grocery store, and possibly even in your home. I personally don't want anything to do with that. And I don't care if the FDA deems something like this to be safe in small amounts. It's not food, it's not good for me, and I don't need it. I'm certainly not going to add any of that to my food that I am making at home. Fresh food please!

We've all heard of trans-fats, right? It's important to understand what they are and also know how to avoid them in your food. They are recognized by the words "hydrogenated" or "partially hydrogenated" oils in your ingredient list. Trans-fats are created by adding hydrogen to liquid vegetable oils to make those oils solid at room temperature, therefore increasing the shelf life of these foods. While that might be great for sales, it's not so great for your health. Trans-fats have been shown to raise your LDL cholesterol (bad cholesterol) and decrease your HDL cholesterol (good cholesterol), thus increasing heart disease risk. They have also been linked to cancer, diabetes, decreased immune function, and more. These fats are EVERYWHERE in processed foods, especially baked goods, snacks and fried food. This is why it is so important to start reading labels.

One of the other big ones to avoid: high fructose corn syrup. HFCS is cheaper than sugar, yet sweeter than sugar, making it a great choice money wise for manufacturers. What they aren't sharing with you, is that HFCS consists of fructose and glucose in a 55-45 ratio in an unbound form. This means it is broken down quite differently than regular sugar... it's even worse. Fructose and glucose are bound together in cane sugar in a 50-50 ratio, making it harder for the body to first break down. Yet the unbound fructose in HFCS goes directly to the liver immediately to be stored as fat, and causing huge insulin spikes. Too much of this on a regular basis can wreak havoc on your liver - potentially causing fatty liver disease. The take away here is, if you see HFCS on the ingredient list on any food you are considering, put it down. It is poor quality processed junk. You don't need that if you're trying to eat well and take care of yourself.

The list goes on and on of other harmful ingredients found in processed foods. Artificial sweeteners, food dyes, artificial flavors, MSG, and a whole slew of other preservatives that we can't pronounce. The more of this we can avoid, the better for our overall health. This is why it is so important to make as much fresh food of your own as you possibly can, and when you HAVE to buy some processed foods, read the labels!!!

Prevent Disease

Every piece of food you choose to put in your mouth on any given day is either causing you harm, or helping you. It's either causing disease, or fighting it. It's either making you fat, or helping you stay fit. It's that simple. We don't realize the damage that we are doing by simply making the wrong choices when it comes to food. Try to start thinking of your food intake in these terms. I'm not suggesting everyone should strive to be perfect from here on out when it comes to eating (I certainly am not), but when you do make a wrong choice, at least recognize it for what it is. When we go through our day with blinders on thinking that certain choices don't really matter, we're just fooling ourselves.

> "Eating crappy food isn't a reward, it's a punishment."
> -Drew Carey

And how about saying "everything in moderation"? Quite honestly, I think it's easy for people to "everything in moderation" themselves to death. The problem here is that moderation means something different to everyone, and it can end up being a catch all excuse for eating junk whenever you feel like it. Moderation to one person may mean eating a piece of cake only after dinner every night. To someone else, eating a piece of cake once per week, or even once per month may be considered moderation. There is no measurement to the word "moderation" and I think it can get people into trouble when they use this as an excuse to eat anything they want, as long as it's not constant. Finding a good sense of moderation in your diet can be very helpful... but you need to be honest with yourself as far as what that really means, and how it is working for you.

When we put food into the two categories I mentioned earlier, it can be helpful. Of the food that is fighting disease and/or keeping you fit, you may have all you want. It's that other category to keep in moderation. The food that is causing disease and/or making you fat, should be limited. This way all of the bad food is grouped together. So you can't say that having cake 3 times a week is okay, because that's moderation... but then also having a soda once per day this week, because that's moderation... and then adding in a donut only on Saturdays and Sundays, because that is moderation. Group all that together, and there is no moderation. It's all in one category and it's too much. They're not separate instances of eating poorly just because they were separate items. Be true to yourself! If you save those things for special parties, birthdays, a certain holiday, etc., then it truly is a special treat, and you can allow yourself the leeway for that occasion without feeling bad.

Low-Carb Diets

Low-carbohydrate diets have become very popular because they tend to be a great way to lose weight and keep it off. A great benefit to eating this way is that we can lower our insulin resistance, which in turn can prevent damage to our blood vessels and possibly heart attack and stroke. Eating a low-carb diet can also decrease your triglyceride levels, increase your HDL (good cholesterol), and possibly decrease your LDL (bad cholesterol). The debate on LDL particles being the benchmark for heart disease goes around and around all the time, but it may be interesting to look at LDL particle size rather than just the number. When LDL particles are large and fluffy, they are known to be heart healthy, as opposed to small LDL particles which are more prevalent in people with heart disease. Eating a low-carb diet has a tendency to create large LDL particles.

Food prep

My number one piece of advice when it comes to food, is make it yourself. Some nurses may complain that they don't have time to make their own food, or it's too hard. I get it. I know we're all busy. Do the best you can with the time you have, but please make an effort for your own sake. Look at our lifestyle these days. Parents are so busy being taxi drivers for all of the 85 activities their children are in, working full time, and balancing all of life's other events.

No wonder drive-thru meals and takeout have become so popular. We've been brainwashed to not have home cooked meals anymore. We've grown accustomed to thinking that this rushed lifestyle is the way it's supposed to be. Well I think it's wrecking everything, right along with our health and fitness. Health aside, how much better for your family life to have everyone sitting down at a table together with fresh, homemade food rather than passing each other in the doorway with a micro-waved Hot Pocket in hand?

Preparing your own fresh food does not mean you have to be all fancy with recipes that have an ingredient list a mile long. Start simple, if this is where you want to be. Start by simply buying fresh veggies to cut up or put in a salad. Or if you prefer, buy frozen veggies if that's easier for you (although I think fresh just tastes so much better!).

Start with small steps. If you're used to buying takeout meals 3 times a week, try cutting it down to once per week. Try making two or three more home cooked meals per week than you're used to. Try swapping out one of your sodas every day for a glass of water instead. Make a conscious effort with these small steps, and continue to progress even more when you feel ready. Remember that each positive small step along the way is a step in the right direction. Progress is still progress, not matter how small, and every small change adds up in the big picture!

> **"Those who think they have no time for healthy eating will sooner or later have to find time for illness."**
> **-Edward Stanley**

A great way to help start the process of more homemade meals and snacks at home is picking one or two days per week when you can set aside a couple of hours at a time and make food in bulk. Pre-make several meals and store them either in your fridge or freezer until you can use them. This can seem like an overwhelming task if you are new to this process, but start small. See how it goes just making a few things ahead of time. Planning your food is huge. Deciding what you are going to eat before the week even starts takes all the last minute guess work out of the stressful mid-week grind. If you know you will be working the next few days, pre-make whatever food you need to bring with you to work. Or if you are one of the many nurses out there who just work weekends, maybe Thursday or Friday is your meal prep day to get things ready for the days ahead.

This is your life saver when it comes to you not relying on whatever the cafeteria has to offer, or falling victim to everyone ordering takeout on a busy weekend (and let's face it... it's usually never something healthy for a takeout order!). If you've already put in all that work to make and bring your food, chances are you are going to eat it. Don't give yourself the option not to. Be in control of your eating by prepping your meals and always being prepared.

Two Ingredient Pancakes

-2 eggs

-1 mostly green banana (not ripe at all!)

Blend together in a blender to mix well; add a dash of cinnamon if desired; cook on stovetop over medium heat in a pan with some ghee (clarified butter) or coconut oil until browned. The key here is using the green banana. If you use one that is too ripe, the pancakes will fall apart and be difficult to flip. I like to multiply this recipe and make a huge batch to keep in the freezer. Top with fresh berries, almond butter and banana slices, raw honey, or some real butter and pure maple syrup!

Have you tried prepping green smoothies for the week? This is super easy and can be a life saver when you're short on time during the week. Get some plastic zip lock freezer bags and fill with the goodies. To each bag, add one banana, a handful of greens (baby spinach, kale, collard greens, Swiss chard, etc), a handful of berries or other fruit (fresh or frozen - I use blueberries or strawberries, pineapple and mango chunks as my favorites) and any other add-ins you wish, like ground flax seed, hemp seed, or chia seeds. Put the bags in the freezer, and take out one at a time when you want a smoothie. Place all ingredients in a blender with one to one and a half cups of water or coconut water (great after a sweaty workout to replace electrolytes!) and blend until smooth. Try it!

Diet Trends

Let's talk for a minute about all the diets we hear thrown around all the time in conversation with those trying to lose weight or make healthier lifestyle changes. First and foremost, I don't care what a diet claims to do for you, if it's not putting its main focus on eating fresh, real food, don't waste your time.

The idea of people doing these "all shakes" types of diets makes me crazy. Okay, is it possible that someone could actually lose weight if they only drank these health shakes for every meal over the next month? Sure! But let's see that person in a few more months time after that plan is done. I can almost guarantee that in just about every case like this, that person will gain back all their weight, and possibly even more. Why? Because that was nothing but a short term fix. A quick plan with an end date. Just suffer through for 30 days of torture, and see the results! Those results that won't last and did you no good over the long run.

And I hate when others see this kind of stuff and ask the question "Does that diet really work?" Or say things like "This one worked for her". Because someone had short term positive results does not make this a good choice. Did it "work" in the short term? Sure. But it only hurts in the long run. The biggest problem here is that diet didn't teach anyone the value of eating fresh whole foods. Drinking shakes at every meal is not sustainable forever. Eventually that person will go back to food... and most likely the same foods that got them overweight and sick in the first place.

Balsamic Turkey Meatballs

-2 lbs organic ground turkey

-1/2 cup diced onion

-2 Tablespoons balsamic vinegar

-1 teaspoon pepper

-2 teaspoons garlic salt

-1 1/2 Tablespoons onion powder

-2 Tablespoons balsamic vinegar

Mix all ingredients together in large bowl. Form balls in your hands and brown on stovetop in a pan heated with 1-2 Tablespoons coconut oil, turning frequently to brown all sides. Once lightly browned, place in crockpot and cook on low for 2-3 hours with your favorite sauce; or place on baking sheet lined with parchment paper and bake at 350 for 15- 20 minutes to cook through.

Now to talk about diets that focus on eating actual food. I must start here by saying one very important thing. As mentioned earlier, WE ARE ALL DIFFERENT!!! While some people thrive on a vegetarian diet, others may feel horribly sick, tired and weak. And on the other hand for those who claim that they feel best on high protein diets with lots of meat, others may not feel well eating a diet containing a lot of meat. While some people insist that giving up gluten is completely necessary to lose weight and feel better, others may do fine with some gluten in their diet and be perfectly healthy and fit. Some claim that giving up dairy is necessary for them to feel better and lose weight. Biochemically, we are all different and have individual needs when it comes to eating. Find what works for YOU!!!

On another note, many people have sensitivities to certain foods and are not even aware that these exact foods are what's causing their problems. We all know people who suffer from bloating, brain fog, GI distress, skin issues, insomnia, headaches or joint pains just to name a few... and many of these symptoms can be related to what they are putting in their mouth. The best way to figure this out is to try an elimination diet, or reset diet if you will. This is a good way to know what foods may be bothering you and possibly hindering your overall health and ability to feel well.

There are many different ways of doing this out there, but for the most part, you would avoid certain foods for thirty days, and then slowly reintroduce foods one at a time and see how they affect you. I like to do this myself at least once or twice a year just to reset myself if I have strayed a bit too far from my normal habits. Things I recommend avoiding during these thirty days: all sugar (and sweeteners of any kind), all grains, all processed foods, dairy, legumes (and peanuts are part of this group), all sodas and fruit juices, and alcohol. If you have any autoimmune problems, you may also want to cut out eggs and nightshade vegetables (tomatoes, eggplant, peppers, potatoes - these can cause inflammation in susceptible people).

So what should you eat? All meat and poultry (organic and free range is best, and try to keep processed meat to a minimum), fish (wild is best, and fatty fish is preferred - salmon, sardines, etc), eggs (if no autoimmune issues) any and all vegetables, fruit, nuts and seeds, black coffee and tea are permitted, but limit to once or twice per day, and plenty of healthy fats like coconut oil, ghee (this is clarified butter without the dairy), and extra virgin olive oil. Doing this for thirty days (without cheating!) can decrease chronic inflammation in your body, increase your energy levels, help regulate blood sugar, burn fat, decrease cravings, improve digestion, and help you identify which foods may be triggering issues in your life.

After the thirty days, you can start reintroducing some of those foods you may have missed, like yogurt or rice for instance. But be sure to only introduce a new food every three days so you know exactly which food is bothering you if you end up having some kind of reaction

(GI upset, bloating, skin irritation, etc). Keep a food journal for this! As always, I would recommend speaking with your doctor before trying any major changes with your diet, especially if you have known health issues.

I personally do best on a mostly paleo/primal type diet of eating lots of fresh vegetables (raw and cooked), meat (preferably beef from grass fed cows, organic chicken, turkey, lamb), eggs (from my own backyard chickens - the best!), lots of fish (wild, not farmed), nuts and seeds, and fresh fruit. I do allow myself some dairy since I do tolerate it well, but I try to limit it to organic raw milk options when possible. Full fat Greek yogurt, raw milk cheese, butter from grass fed cows (or ghee) and kefir are a few of my favorites. I have not ventured to trying drinking raw milk itself, but the little milk I do have (a tiny splash in my coffee) is organic whole milk. Okay, and ice cream. Yes ice cream on a limited basis. I am human and will allow myself things that make me very happy from time to time that may not be on the "healthy" list, and that's okay, but I do need to keep it in check.

I do best when I stay away from things made from wheat. I just feel better without it. For years I would love my big chewy bagel every morning, and not realizing that was adding to my brain fog, bloating, lethargy and sugar crash later in the day. And let me just warn any of you who think you'll instantly be healthy by buying every "gluten free" box of processed food on the shelf. No. If you want to avoid gluten, eat more natural foods that don't contain gluten. While some of these store options are okay, the majority of your diet should not consist of this stuff.

What you eat 80-90% of the time is what matters, so don't beat yourself up, or judge someone else for straying off the "healthy" list every now and again. It's your body, and your choice. Don't be a slave to food, or make yourself feel imprisoned by how you eat. Once you start eating more fresh food and less processed food, you will feel so much better and hopefully want to continue on that path because you enjoy it. But life happens around us as well. Do what works for you and fits into your lifestyle, and don't beat yourself up with a pity party every time a small mishap occurs. Focus on what you are doing 80-90% of the time and be proud of that. Any positive move in the right direction is still progress. Celebrate the small victories and little changes you make over time. It all adds up!

Eating Patterns

This is a topic that varies widely among so many health and fitness experts. We've all heard the lines before - "eat at the same times every day", "eat small frequent meals every 2 hours", "never eat past 7 p.m.", "eat a small snack before bed to keep your metabolism burning", "never skip a meal", "ALWAYS eat breakfast everyday". Now while I'm not going to say any of these are necessarily wrong, I am going to say a few things about why these can cause problems. When we fix ourselves on the idea of a strict pattern that must be followed with our eating, then what happens to us on those days that for some crazy reason you just can't make it happen? That's it. You're toast. Might as well throw in the towel and give up, because you screwed everything up and now it won't work. At this point, just wait until next January 1st and start all over again. We stress out if we weren't able to get in our 10 a.m. snack that was all planned out and had to happen to stick to the rules.... or you slept late and didn't have time to make your breakfast before leaving for work... or you were invited to dinner at a friend's house and they served things long after your "cut-off" time of 7 p.m. ... or you just had a crazy busy shift at work and you are not able to eat at the exact time that you had planned to stick to your plan (yeah, like almost every day for a nurse... right?). Then we freak out if we ever stray away from the plan, because "the plan" is what's going to make or break my weight loss and overall health. No. It's not. While trying to have some structure with your eating most of the time, we need to allow ourselves a little grace when it actually isn't going to happen. And honestly, this can be a blessing.

Let's discuss the topic of intermittent fasting. WHAT? This can be a bit mind blowing for some people to grasp, but hear me out. What if you actually did skip a meal every now and then? What if you DIDN'T eat breakfast all the time? What if you were in a fasted state for up to 18 hours a day and ate all your food in a 6-8 hour window instead of spread all throughout the day? You would live. And it actually could be beneficial! Mark Sisson mentions in The Primal Blueprint that you could actually reprogram your genes to burn more fat by doing this, and the whole process can possibly be good for your overall health by promoting insulin sensitivity, helping decrease body fat and oxidative damage, along with lowering blood pressure. That sounds great to me! Studies have shown that your body is actually most sensitive to insulin following a period of fasting, thus helping your body use the food it does consume much more efficiently.

Peanut Butter Protein Cookies

-1 egg

-1 1/2 cup natural organic peanut butter (chunky preferred)

-1/3 cup pure maple syrup

-1 1/2 teaspoon vanilla extract

-1/2 cup Bob's Red Mill whey protein powder

-1/4 cup ground flaxseed

Add all ingredients together in a bowl and mix well. Form 15-18 into balls in your hands and place on a greased cookie sheet. Bake at 325 for 10-12 minutes, or until edges are slightly golden brown. Let cool 5-10 minutes before removing from pan.

There are many different ways it can be done. Some people do it as mentioned above with eating all their calories for the day within a 6-8 hour period and fasting for the remaining 16-18 hours. Others may do a one day per week planned fast that goes on for a full 24-36 hours. Or some may just decide to skip a meal when they realize they just truly aren't hungry at a time they had planned to eat.... I think this is my favorite! Listening to your body is my number one take away rule for all things health and fitness.

The 5/2 plan is another popular idea. For this plan, twice per week you would eat only 2 meals per day, trying to keep those meals in the ballpark of around 500-600 calories each. You could spread those days out to do this maybe on Mondays and Thursdays let's say. The other five days per week you would eat your normal three meals. This plan helps you to cut calories intermittently which is easier to accomplish rather than maintaining a lower caloric intake on a daily basis. You could potentially cut 1,000 - 3,000 calories per week with this plan, which in turn would lead to weight loss over time. This is much more practical and sustainable rather than trying to do it all in a straight line.

> "Mindful eating replaces self-criticism with self-nurturing. It replaces shame with respect for your own inner wisdom."
> -Jan Chozen Bays

If you think about it, we don't go all-out in the gym every day, seven days per week. Workouts should be somewhat cyclical. We have our heavy days and our lighter days for recovery. Why not use this method of thinking with our eating as well? It only makes sense. We could save our heavy lifting days for the days we know we will be eating more, and our recovery or lighter days can be on the days we eat less. This concept of using periodization with your eating AND workouts can be a total game changer for your health and weight loss goals.

So which is it? Do we need to cut calories in order to lose weight, or does quality of calories matter more than quantity? Actually, it is a little bit of both. Somewhere in the middle is where the magic is. Using fasting to cut calories will not compensate for an otherwise horrible diet. You may have heard the phrase "you can't out exercise a bad diet", and this is pretty much true. The quality of your calories matter. Some foods your body will burn off quicker and more efficiently, and other foods will be stored directly as fat along with making you feel sluggish, lazy and unable to have any productive kind of workout. Processed foods, especially, tend to be a lot easier to over consume than fresh food. Be careful! That being said, of course you can certainly over eat and gain weight with eating too much of the right kinds of foods every day. If you're taking in more than you are burning off, even if it's healthy food, you will eventually end up with weight gain. Therefore, it is definitely necessary to have some sort of caloric deficit to achieve weight loss.

Do you ever truly pay attention to when you are actually hungry and when you're not? People who get into regimented eating schedules usually do not, and often end up eating out of habit or routine when your body may actually not need or want food at that time. We sometimes "schedule" ourselves to death and end up working against our own goals. Now what MAY happen if you first try to just skip a meal is that, yes, you are hungry and then you're mad. Why? Because you have trained your body to want and expect food at certain times with your habits (and especially if you are custom to eating a high carbohydrate diet, that angry sugar crash can be nasty).

What I have found with myself is that after a few times of trying to work through this (while also making sure I clean up my eating by eliminating simple carbohydrates and sugar), my body has actually acclimated pretty well to this process. I do not do this all the time, but occasionally (pretty much like the 5/2 plan). What I love the most is that this can provide some freedom from the everyday grind. It's less to prepare and think about in any given day, and can honestly be a great time and money saver. However, please consider discussing this with your physician (especially if you have any significant health issues like Diabetes, etc) before trying anything like this. Wait, nurses already know that, right? Of course.

Chapter 5

Exercise for the Nurse

Ha! This is the fun part... at least for me. Being able to exercise is a privilege. Do you know that? Do you realize the gift that it truly is? Most people do not, based on how dreaded they make it sound, or treat it as a punishment rather than something they should feel blessed to be able to do. All I have to say to put this into perspective, is think of someone who is UNABLE to exercise, even if they wanted to. Think of a paraplegic. Think of those with horrible chronic pain or debilitating disease. Think of emaciated bed ridden elderly people who can't move at all for themselves. Guess what they would probably give anything to do? They would love the ability to go get some exercise... but they can't. They don't have that as an option. It just won't happen for them. So how do we sit here as able bodied people and dare complain about physical activity? It is a gift. Treat is as such, and do it for those who cannot. Or better yet, do it for yourself because you ARE able. You have that gift at your finger tips. Treasure that!

You could argue that as nurses we get a ton of physical activity on any given day whether it be from walking 10,000 steps in one shift, or lifting heavy patients or equipment. I get that, but it's not purposeful exercise in it's true meaning. Nursing is for sure an extremely physical job, but I would not quite call that a healthy dose of exercise in the true sense. Our bodies need to move in an organized manner with a purpose rather than in unorganized spurts that catch us off guard at work and potentially cause injury when our bodies are not strong enough or conditioned enough to handle it. When we add organized exercise to our life making us stronger and more efficient with our movement, this makes those unorganized spurts we encounter at work all that more bearable. This is why it is crucial for nurses especially to get exercise outside of work. Preventing injury and keeping your body strong and able to move well for the rest of your life is the goal here.

Let's start by mentioning some of the many benefits of getting regular exercise. How about increasing your mood for starters? I don't know about you, but this is one of my very favorite benefits of exercise. It's a happy pill without taking a pill! For real. Exercise has been proven to be extremely effective in treating depression... in some cases even more so than prescription medications. That's a huge benefit that is so underused by so many. I bet you can think of a few grouchy and depressed people who could benefit from that... or maybe it's you. When we get a good dose of exercise, our body releases those little chemicals called endorphins. Endorphins trigger a positive feeling in the body, and can even be addictive. I don't know about you, but I would say that's a pretty great thing to start being addicted to. I know I am, and it is so true. If you don't know this yourself, I bet you know someone who gets so mad and frustrated when they miss a workout because they miss that feeling. That natural "high" it produces that becomes so addictive. What a beautiful thing. Endorphins are also natural analgesics that can reduce the perception of pain. Again, awesome!!! Exercise, or take a pain pill... depending on the reason for pain of course, I think exercise wins here. I'm all for a natural remedy over taking a pill any day.

How about lifting your energy level? Sounds kind of crazy, but when you expend more energy with exercise, it actually gives you an energy boost to better perform your other daily tasks. What a gift! What nurse couldn't use a little extra energy boost to get through a difficult twelve hour shift? Or how about trying to make it through a night shift? Now that's tough, and yes, exercise can help here. Not only can it give you a physical energy boost, but a mental one as well. Exercise can help you feel more alert, and even help improve your memory!

Now for improving your sleep. I know this is very true for myself. When I am exercising regularly, I am definitely sleeping better. No doubt. I know that if there is ever a week where life gets too crazy and I just can't squeeze in any exercise at all, I am not sleeping as soundly as usual for sure. It's so easy to spot this out, at least for me. If you are someone who struggles with getting quality sleep, and you are not currently exercising on a routine basis, I would definitely recommend giving it a try!

Let's mention disease prevention for a moment. Again, as nurses we see it all... and it's ugly out there. We come across one horrible situation after another on a daily basis, and sometimes it's just plain scary. We KNOW that exercise helps prevent many diseases. We KNOW what we need to do. But are we doing it? Or are we going to be left to be one of those patients we see so often with medical issues that could have easily been prevented with regular exercise and self care? NO! Please don't do it. We know that regular exercise can boost your immunity, decrease your risk for heart disease, diabetes, many different kinds of cancers, and

> "Some people want it to happen, some wish it would happen, others make it happen."
> -Michael Jordan

more. Your life is precious. Enjoy it to the fullest and don't let preventable diseases take away your freedom and enjoyment. You deserve better, and you can do better. Not to mention, you have a much better chance of increasing your life expectancy and live longer than if you were not exercising.

And now for the obvious reasons of increasing strength and flexibility. Nurses do a lot of heavy lifting on any given day. That's a fact. From lifting heavy patients, pushing stretchers or beds, moving equipment and so much more, nurses use a lot of muscle power every day! Just think of how much better prepared you could be to handle those tasks if you were doing some sort of strength training outside of work. When your muscles are strong and used to being pushed in a controlled fashion on a regular basis with exercise, they will be that much more able to handle the unexpected at work. You will carry yourself taller, have better posture and just be stronger over all in performing whatever is required of you. This will certainly help decrease your potential for injury on the job.

We've all heard horror stories of nurses who have gotten seriously injured on the job from some sort of physical situation that got the best of them. Some of these instances end with very serious long term debilitations that are just devastating. This breaks my heart, and it's scary. Being a nurse is great, but wrecking your life with a debilitating injury is not cool. Building muscle strength outside of work is your best defense against this situation. No one wants to see that happen. We lose a certain percentage of muscle mass every year past the age of thirty unless we are actively trying to keep it by doing some resistance training. Don't let your muscle waste away, and in turn leave you with a body that is unprepared to handle the unexpected on any given day.

We can't forget another big one here - weight loss. Yes, of course, regular exercise will help with weight loss. This is probably the #1 reason so many people do get into exercise, and it certainly can be effective in that area. But then there are always those people who would much rather take a "quick-fix" pill to lose the weight because then they don't have to do all that hard work with exercise. Good luck with that. Not only do you risk dangerous side effects with any type of weight loss pill, but you are missing out on all the other health benefits of exercise that are (in my opinion) even more important than just losing a few pounds. Exercise is always a better choice. DO THE WORK. On the other side of hard work, comes great rewards. There is no easy out for lazy people. Sorry.

So let's see, you could improve your mood, potentially beat (or greatly improve) depression, have more energy, sleep better, prevent deadly and debilitating diseases, improve your overall strength and flexibility which could greatly improve your total quality of life, and (the big favorite) lose some unwanted weight. I personally don't see a downside here. You just can't argue this and win for the other side (although people sure do try).

> "Excuses are lies wrapped up in reason."
> -Howard Wright

And why is it that people fight this? We can wrap that up in one word: excuses. That's all it is. I know everyone has their own sob story of how they just can't find the time to exercise... or they can't afford a gym membership... or they are too tired from being on their feet all day at their job... or they don't know what to do at the gym so they just don't do anything. The list goes on and on and on. If you are serious about your health, and you truly want to improve in all those areas above, you will make it happen. Someone else reading this right now is busier than you, and they are making the time to exercise. It might not be at the ideal time they would choose, or using the exact equipment they wish they had, or in the perfect setting with the world's best trainer. They're just getting it done however, wherever, and whenever they can... because they make it a priority. That's the difference here.

Show me how you spend your time and money, and I will tell you what your priorities are in life. It really is that simple. People have no problem buying fancy clothes or paying to get their nails done every week, but those same people will cringe at paying for a gym membership or a trainer. Your body is the best investment you have. Spend some time and money to make it last and function well.

You're not exempt from all this because of whatever reason you can throw at me. I've heard them all, and unless you are physically incapable of moving, then you can exercise. If you're not willing to make some uncomfortable sacrifices to make it happen, then you're really not serious enough about your own health and well-being at all. Think about that. You are the only one holding you back. No one else can do that. We are only confined by the walls we build around ourselves. Sometimes we are our own worst enemies. Get past your own self and get on with life!

Resistance Training

Resistance training (or strength training) is such a misunderstood topic among many women. First of all, resistance training simply means exercises that cause resistance on a muscle to make it stronger. This does not have to include using weights. There are plenty of body weight exercises that can work wonders for a great muscle building workout. You can also use resistance bands or tubing, and then of course dumbbells, barbells, kettlebells, etc. People who think of themselves as big to begin with tend to shy away from any type of resistance training in fear that it will make them appear "bulky". This is a myth, and it needs to be squashed. When you build muscle in your body, you actually become tighter, leaner and potentially smaller than you were before. Five pounds of muscle is much more firm and compact than five pounds of fat. That is for sure.

In fact, many women find that once they begin resistance training they actually don't need to lose any weight at all. They may be much happier with their entire physique simply because of a better body composition (ratio of muscle to fat). Men, on the other hand, will grow much larger from weight training than women, and this is because men have a lot more testosterone than women. And if you're going to ask about massive women with huge muscles you've seen in magazines, this is so far above and beyond what the average female is doing with weight training. Way beyond. Not to worry.

So let's explore some of the other benefits of resistance training. Did you know that it actually takes more calories to maintain muscle than fat? That's a bonus! You can actually create a better metabolism when you have more muscle. I'm all for that, because I like to eat. And I will tell you from personal experience, I am always much more hungry on days that I lift heavy than on days that I don't. You might think that's a bad thing to just eat more, but you can actually create such a huge calorie burn from lifting weights that you simply are able to eat that much more to replenish what you just burned off. But don't take that as an open invitation to stuff yourself with junk. That's not the point here. By all means if you're really ravenous, eat a bit more on those days, but make sure it is good food that will help your muscles repair and build back up to be ready for the next time.

Try to always include some form of protein after a good resistance training session to help in that muscle rebuilding. I love the saying "muscles are torn down in the gym, fed in the kitchen and built up in bed". All three parts are equally important in growing stronger. Did you ever think about the fact that you are actually creating small micro tears in your muscles when we are performing any weight training exercises? This is actually not where the muscle growth happens. For many hours after your workout, the body then works hard to repair and adapt the muscle to better be able to handle that same stimulus in the future. Choosing proper nutrition is extremely important in helping that muscle repair itself.

And then rest! This is where the muscle growth happens. How much quality rest you get can have just as much effect on your muscle building ability. It is a misconception to think that you need to constantly be training to build the most muscle. Weight training increases your production of growth hormone which helps with muscle growth, yet over training can actually decrease the amount of growth hormone produced, in turn hurting your progress. Over training can actually halt your progress, so take your rest days and get enough sleep. Growth hormone is secreted at night when we are sleeping as well. This secretion often occurs at a higher rate during the first part of the night, making it a good idea to get to bed on the earlier side rather than later. When we go short on sleep, we can actually blunt the effect of growth hormone, thus limiting our recovery and muscle growth ability. Get your rest!

Why not do some strength training for the obvious reason - to just be strong! Increasing your overall strength is such an awesome feeling. It makes everyday life so much easier. As nurses, we lift all day long. We lift heavy patients, heavy equipment, push heavy beds and much more. Why not build some muscle so you can lift things like a boss without giving it a second thought? Why should you need to ask for help all the time to carry anything heavy? Forget that. Increase your strength and lift it yourself! Being strong enough to handle these situations safely can instantly decrease your risk of injury, especially on the job. When your body is strong, the muscles, tendons and ligaments are much less likely to give way under stress. I would rather be prepared for the unexpected and bounce back easily rather than risk getting hurt because I lack the strength needed for whatever comes my way. What a liberating feeling that is to not have to rely on someone else (or a GUY) all the time to have to move anything heavy for you. Of course, there are times it is just safer to have help along side of you, and by all means ask for help when it's necessary. But to make yourself stronger for those smaller tasks, it can be such a great feeling. Your everyday tasks will become a breeze.

And not to mention, talk about a confidence boost! What an awesome feeling it is to know that you worked hard to become stronger and, in turn, now have so many more freedoms to enjoy and activities to perform in life that you once may have shied away from. You will stand taller, walk with more confidence in your stride, and take on life with a whole new outlook. Most people underestimate the effect weight training can have on their overall self-esteem. When you challenge yourself to lift heavy and push yourself past limits you thought you had, that can honestly shoot your confidence through the roof. You become very proud of what you accomplished. This can change your entire outlook on other challenges in life. When you realize you CAN do what you thought you could NOT do in a physical sense, this can carry over into other areas of your life. Being dedicated to strength training and seeing the positive results can help you be more dedicated in other areas of your life as well.

Hey, the sky is the limit! No one can hold you back, except for you. Seeing the positive mental effects with weight training can push you to become more determined to succeed in so much more. It can give you that drive to push harder, be more determined to go after what you want, and just plain feels awesome. Go get some of that. It's such a gift!

Many of us worry as we get older about bone loss. I know plenty of people (and you probably do too) who are taking all kinds of supplements to help prevent bone loss. No one wants to risk breaking an arm or a hip from a fall as we get older. Strength training can help prevent bone loss, and over time, possibly even help build new bone. A good strength training routine done at least two to three times per week can greatly increase your bone density, making the risk of fractures or breaks that much lower. The way to make something stronger is to put some stress on it and force it to resist that pressure. This is what happens to our bones with resistance training, and it's so important. Just one of the many examples of a situation where a medication can potentially be avoided altogether simply by taking care of yourself in the right way. This is one of my major take away points for this book - when we take care of ourselves first, we decrease the need for medications and disease treatment.

What does weight training do for overall disease prevention? Probably a lot more than you think. Lifting weights can increase your HDL (good cholesterol) and decrease your LDL (bad cholesterol) making your lipid profile look so much better and make your doctor happy! It can lower your blood pressure and decrease your risk of heart disease. Your body will become more sensitive to insulin, making your risk for Diabetes much lower. You can decrease your risk of certain cancers (like breast cancer) and just plain boost your overall immunity to fighting off colds and illness in general.

These all sound like more good reasons to lift weights in my opinion. And within that long list, are many more opportunities to avoid taking unnecessary medications (meds for Diabetes, high blood pressure, cholesterol lowering drugs, cold medicine, and let's just say any cancer treatments that can be avoided - need I say more). Just say no to drugs, right? When they can be avoided, absolutely. I'll take exercise and eating right any day over a long list of pills to take every day that all have potentially dangerous side effects.

Do you ever listen to those drug commercials on television? Everyone is smiling looking like they're having the time of their life with these medications, and then you hear the horrifying list of side effects blurted out as a side note. Unbelievable! I would be terrified to take half of these pills based on that. It's scary! And many of them even have death on that list. Wake up people!!! Why ignore taking care of yourself the natural way just to take nasty meds that cost a lot and can potentially cause you so much harm??? This is where I get angry. Everything is about money out there, and the drug companies want to make lots of it.

It sounds all great to come up with these quick fixes to your health problems, yet how many doctors out there are actually pushing healthy eating and a sensible exercise program FIRST before talking about medications? Not enough, that's for sure. Don't be steamrolled into that thinking that you need to take every drug suggested to you. The bottom line is that someone somewhere is trying to make money off of that. Use some common sense first, take care of your body the way you were meant to first, THEN see if medications are necessary at that point.

One of my absolute favorite reasons of all for lifting weights is for the emotional and psychological benefits. Lifting heavy weights just feels GOOD. It gives this crazy boost of energy like I've never known. It's powerful. It's invigorating. It's just plain "bad-ass" if I can say that! Something happens inside that takes away all doubt, insecurity, worry, fear or anger when you lift. Feeling down on yourself? Go lift. Feeling angry? Go lift. Feeling insecure and not good enough? Go lift. All those doubts and bad feelings are replaced with this awesome feeling of strength and confidence that just overpowers everything else. It really is that awesome. And if you've never experienced how healing that is, then you are missing out.

By far, the best lifting sessions I ever had have been on days that I am angry or frustrated at someone else. Take all that adrenaline and all those nasty thoughts out in a lifting session, and you will be amazed at your strength on those days! And suddenly, you're not mad any more. Instead, your proud of yourself. You feel powerful and accomplished. Your confidence is through the roof. You stand taller and forget what you were even mad about in the first place (okay, maybe). This is such a healing and therapeutic way to deal with stress and other difficult emotions rather than so many other destructive options that are out there.

Again with another reference to avoiding medication here. Side effects of medications, as we've already mentioned, can be disastrous. But hey - what are the side effects of lifting weights and getting exercise? Oh, that would be looking better, feeling better, being happier, less anxious, less risk of disease, being stronger, having a better metabolism, more energy, sleeping better, and greater self esteem. I don't see one negative in there. And before someone says "you could get hurt", really? I would rather get hurt lifting weights at the gym (that I would most likely recover from if I was training properly) than wasting my life on a couch being out of shape and possibly destroying my life much MORE from all kinds of medical problems because I didn't want to get hurt lifting weights. Not to mention, the weights won't hurt you. It's how you use the weights that will hurt you. Learn the right way, use good form, and you will be much less likely to get hurt. Plus, we could get hit by a bus on any given day. Are you never going to leave your house because of that? Life itself is full of ways to get hurt. Don't stay away from the ones with the greatest benefit to yourself in fear of getting hurt. Think about how much sense that really makes. Not much.

There are so many great ways to get these benefits. If you have never used equipment before in weight training, by all means start out with body weight movements first to be sure your form is good before using any equipment (and you may not ever want to add equipment - and that's okay!).

Start out with body weight squats, planks, and push up progressions before using weights. When trying to squat, place your feet shoulder width apart (or a little wider if that's more comfortable for you), plant your heels firmly into the ground (toes may point outward slightly), and lower down into the squat position keeping your back as straight as possible. Do not let your heels come off the ground or round your back. Push back up through your heels (not the balls of your feet!) to a standing position. Some people can get down to a really low squat, and others may not be able to go below parallel. Get to where you can. Us nurses usually have to squat down multiple times a day on the job, especially in an ICU- type -setting (where I've spent most of my career) emptying Foley catheters, measuring chest tube outputs and other various drains. Doing this every hour for a twelve hour shift is a lot of squatting, so make sure your form is good and think about how you lower yourself down and get back up. Once I started squatting at the gym, I started paying much more attention to how I squatted to do things at work, or even at home. Make it a workout, and use good form!

Try doing planks every day and see if you can hold them longer each time (even if only for a few seconds). Try them up on your hands, and also on your elbows for a variation. After you get better at planks, try some pushup progressions. Pushups are a fantastic body weight exercise, and yes you can do them! If this seems impossible to you, start with wall pushups. Then progress to a bench, and then finally to the ground. Start with one. The more you do them, the better you will get, and you will reap the rewards of strong arms, a strong core, and better total upper body definition.

Benefits of Planks

Planks create a strong core. They engage your rectus abdominis, transverse abdominis, obliques, and glutes. Strengthening these muscles can help you lift more weight safely, improve performance in sports, and prevent injury. Your core is the foundation to all movement. Keep it strong so you will move well! Not to mention, you will gain upper body strength the longer you are able to hold the position.

Forearm or Straight-Arm Plank:
Go down onto your forearms (or hands keeping arms straight) with legs extended back. Keep elbows directly under shoulders. Come up onto the balls of your feet and keep your spine straight. Draw your belly button up towards your spine and hold for 30 seconds to start.

Side Plank:
Come onto your right hand or forearm with elbow under shoulder and feet stacked. Keep your hip lifted so you make a straight line from your head to your feet. Keep core engaged the entire time and hold for 30 seconds each side.

Practice the hip hinge movement for your dead lifts before picking up any objects. This is different from a squat! Watch videos online to see the difference, or have a trainer show you. Learning how to dead lift properly is a great skill to have in all areas of life. When done right, you will protect your back and make a super strong core. You will want to make sure you have a stable core and are able to keep your core stable through certain movements to be sure you are safe when moving on to using equipment. Your core is the foundation of all movement. Make sure you engage your core with any and all types of weight lifting exercises. Pay attention to your hips as well. Are your hips in a neutral position? Or are the tilted forward making your lower back curve and your butt stick out? Try to tuck your tailbone under a bit to correct this. Your posture is so important in weight lifting for best results and to reduce your chance of injury.

My personal favorites for using equipment are barbells and kettlebells. Performing dead lifts, squats, and over head presses with a barbell is a great feeling. You don't have to go super heavy with this either, although I do love heavy lifting. Actually, most people can usually lift a lot heavier than they think. Finding out you are stronger than you thought you were is a pretty cool feeling. I know I shocked myself a few times when I started out lifting, and that's kind of fun. It's almost as if this other part of me shows up that I didn't know was in there when I pick up a heavy barbell. I honestly love that. The key here is to make sure you are using proper form and always have someone coaching you properly if you are not experienced at this. Using proper form is key when it comes to avoiding injury. It's a must.

Using kettlebells for weight training is just awesome. You can use a kettlebell for lots of the same exercises you can do using a dumbbell as well, although I really love the more specific kettlebell exercises such as the swing, for instance. The kettlebell swing is one of the most effective exercises you can do, although it is probably one of the most improperly performed exercises out there. It is a hip hinge exercise, not a squat (be sure to learn the difference before trying this!). Start out by practicing a kettlebell deadlift before moving onto the swing. These are both hip hinge movements, and starting out with the deadlift will be a good precursor before going onto the ballistic movement of the swing. The kettlebell swing is such a powerful exercise for your entire posterior chain. The power for this exercise comes from the hips, not the arms, which is so misunderstood so often. This is not a movement where you are trying to "lift" the kettlebell with your arms! Power comes from the hips here.

> "The kettlebell is an ancient Russian weapon against weakness."
> -Pavel Tsatsouline

The swing can improve your overall strength along with endurance. It can be a super calorie burner to torch fat in a pretty short amount of time. I'm all for achieving more in less time, and I bet most nurses would agree. I also love the fact that with just one kettlebell, you can perform so many different entire body workouts with just one piece of equipment. No gym required! I have my own assortment of kettlebells in my home for days that I cannot get out to the gym for this very reason. They are certainly not some super fancy looking piece of workout equipment, but wow, are they an effective tool for getting the job done. They are super portable, don't take up much space, and don't require a long period of time to get a super effective workout.

Apart from the swing, there are so many other awesome exercises to do with a kettlebell. Turkish get-ups, over head presses, cleans, snatches, figure 8's, lunges with a kettlebell, farmers carries, overhead carries, and the list just goes on. But please get proper training in how to do these moves before just trying on your own. Are kettlebells in and of themselves dangerous? No. How you use the kettlebell is what can be dangerous. As with any exercise equipment, please learn how to properly use it before trying things on your own without proper instruction.

Using a kettlebell for all these exercises is also a great way to improve your grip strength. How strong your grip is actually says a lot about your overall strength. The wide handle on a kettlebell does more for improving your grip strength than holding onto a smaller bar or dumbbell that isn't as thick. The more of your hand you can engage in gripping, the greater your grip strength will increase. Increasing your grip strength will also help greatly if you want to succeed in doing pull-ups at some point. And pull-ups are a phenomenal weight training exercise! Don't be afraid of them. They don't come easy to most people, but with patience and a lot of practice, they can be achieved. Using resistance bands to do assisted pull-ups, and also using rings or TRX bands to do upright rows are two great ways to practice for eventually achieving your first unassisted pull-up.

Dumbbells are also small, portable and easy to use anywhere for resistance training. They are obviously great for upper body exercises, but also great for adding resistance to lower body exercises as well. Squats, lunges (front, back and side), step-ups, dead lifts and calf raises are all examples of lower body exercises that can be accentuated using dumbbells for resistance. There are so many different variations of all of these exercises as well, that it's almost impossible to get bored.

If you're not one of those lucky people to have a full home gym in your own house, you will most likely have to go to a gym to use barbells. Barbells are best used for heavy weight training. When I started lifting with barbells, I feel that it was honestly one of the best things I've ever done. It just feels powerful to lift a bar with whatever weight is appropriate for you - and sometimes that means just the bar- and that's okay! The advantage here is that it gives the possibility of unlimited progression, because you can always add more weight to the bar.

Heavy lifting is great, but be aware that you can also dangerously compress your joints if your workouts are not planned correctly and you are not doing enough off-setting with exercises that actively decompress the joints and help release tension. This is a must if you plan on lifting heavy, and will help prevent injury in the long run. Trust me, I have learned the hard way on this issue. One example of this is to hang from a horizontal bar (pull-up bar if available) to decompress the spine. Also doing forward bends after a squatting session is helpful (place your hands on the floor while keeping your legs stiff at the knees). If you have never used a bar before, please consult with a trainer before trying on your own to be sure you are using proper form. NEVER rush through a warm up session, especially before doing heavy lifts. If you do, you will regret it. Dead lifts, over head presses, front squats, back squats, cleans, snatches and thrusters are just powerful lifts to learn and help build muscle along with amazing confidence. Of course, barbells are not as portable as kettlebells or dumbbells, but if you have the opportunity to use them, it's worth giving it a try. Heavy lifting may not be for everyone, but you don't know until you try. You just might love it - I did!

Think of strength training as just that... training to increase your strength. Training, verses working out, can be a better way to look at this. Don't hurt yourself or abuse equipment trying to rush this too quickly in the name of a good workout. Training is a skill. Something we learn and improve on. Don't go into strength training focusing on merely how many calories you need to burn or how many total reps you could fit in that day. It's so much more than that. And don't always train to exhaustion, but rather leave a little bit left in the tank.

There's a mindset out there that if you're not throwing up or in the fetal position on the floor at the end of your session, then you didn't do it right. Not so. That might sound tough and all, but in all honesty, it's stupid. Unless you are training to be a Navy Seal, there really isn't much need for that kind of torture. I'm all for working hard and pushing myself, but always leave a little something left. What if you get jumped when you leave the gym! You better have some fight left in you!

I know there may still be some skeptics out there. Nurses might say that weightlifting really doesn't apply to them. Sure, you don't NEED to deadlift, but you should be able to safely pick up a heavy piece of equipment (or even a patient) off the floor. You don't

NEED to squat, but getting yourself up and down easily from measuring catheter output, chest tube drainage, or even getting up and down from your chair is certainly helpful. You don't NEED to do Turkish getups, but being able to get yourself up off the floor gracefully even into your old age is certainly a plus. You don't NEED to do lunges, but improving your balance and coordination at work and in life is a great benefit to all. These movements aren't just for body builder muscle heads. They are for nurses. They are for everyone, in everyday life. We all do these types of movements every day, whether we realize it or not. So why not practice them safely and effectively in a workout routine so you are better prepared for the real life situations, therefore making real life easier?

Cardio

Cardiovascular exercise is actually any exercise that raises your heart rate. People greatly misunderstand what it means to do enough "cardio" in their exercise routine. So many of us automatically think of running when we say cardio. By no means is running the only way to get a good elevation in your heart rate with exercise, yet people feel obligated to get on the dreaded treadmill and pound out some miles all for the sake of getting enough cardio. STOP! If you hate running, don't run. There is no need.

First, let's break it down into two topics. There is low-moderate level aerobic exercise which is those long drawn out times of low-moderate intensity for things such as a long brisk walk, a hike or a slow jog. This type of movement is beneficial to our everyday living because it keeps us moving. There is a need for that! If you are someone who has been very sedentary up to this point, a nice brisk walk is a great place for you to start. It is a common mistake for some to think that they need to jump right into some vigorous exercise routine right away when they've been told to start exercising.

If the only movement they have on a regular basis is getting up from the couch and going to the kitchen, then they need to start with 15-20 minute walks a few times per week before doing anything else, and there is nothing wrong with that. It's the right thing to do. Frequent movement at a comfortable pace is necessary and good for all of us. Even those who train hard and have super intense cardio sessions within their routine (we will get more into this in a minute) also need times of a slow and comfortable pace.

Overtraining and over taxing our bodies can be, and is, a serious problem for many. When we push too hard for too many sessions per week, we stress the "fight-or-flight" response that our bodies use in emergencies. Thus secreting more cortisol and potentially causing adrenal fatigue. This can cause a host of problems like decreased immune function, decreased energy level, and overall "burnout". Balancing the tough sessions with some long and drawn out comfortable pace movement is a great way to counteract this and keep things in check. However, that being said, if you're goals are weight loss and/or trying to train for an event, you may need more than just this, eventually.

Now to focus on the more intense cardio sessions. Getting your heart rate really up there to the point of being breathless (in a controlled sense, not short of breath from going past the point of safety) is very beneficial in many ways. We've all heard of HIIT training, right? That's High Intensity Interval Training which involves short bursts of all out effort and then resting briefly to regain your breath and heart rate recovery. Short sprints are an excellent example here. These types of exercises release human growth hormone and testosterone which are helpful in muscle growth, increasing energy levels, and even minimizing the effects of aging. I'll take it! Short bursts of high intensity can train your fast twitch muscles to go even faster the next time. This is super helpful when training for a sporting event or even just increasing your overall ability to outrun your kid. Ha!

And if you hate sprints because you hate running, there are many other options. I love doing 30-45 second intervals of all different drills for some high intensity cardio. Some of my favorite choices are burpees, jump squats, speed skaters, high knees, high speed jump rope, jumping lunges and some quick feet agility drills using an agility ladder. Short bursts, high intensity, short recovery time, and hit it again. The more often you do this the better your recovery time will get, and thus increasing your cardiovascular health. This will also make those longer, less intense cardiovascular exercises seem even easier.

Fat burning is a huge benefit here. The more high intensity exercise you can do, the higher you raise your heart rate, and therefore more calories are burned. And what about after burn! You actually continue burning more calories after this type of workout is done. Extra bang for your buck.

You may have heard somewhere along the line about staying in the "fat burning zone" for your heart rate. I can remember doing workout videos when I was younger and they just kept repeating how important it was to stay in the fat burning zone. I mean, why not? Everyone wants to burn fat, right? What exactly does that mean? Let's break it down. At rest, your body is using primarily all fat as fuel, not carbohydrates. As exercise intensity increases, the ratio changes to using more carbohydrates than fat as the primary fuel. So it has been said to keep your intensity lower to burn a higher percentage of fat calories. While this statement is somewhat true, we need to look at the fact that a higher intensity workout has the ability to burn more overall calories, despite the ratio now being a higher percentage of carbohydrates being burned. So while you could have a higher percentage of fat calories burned during a lower intensity workout, you could burn a larger total number of fat calories with a higher intensity workout, thus making this a better option for ultimately burning the most fat. It is the total number of calories burned that will determine weight loss, not necessarily the source of those calories. Interesting tip. If losing fat is your main goal, don't leave out the high intensity workouts as long as they are safe for you to do.

And just to point out, you can have a cardiovascular effect from doing workouts that are not exactly planned as "cardio". For instance, I know I get my heart rate up pretty high on many kettlebell workouts that I do. That's why I love working out with kettlebells. I feel like you can get it all done at once. Clearly you are getting the strength component, and also a definite cardiovascular benefit from getting your heart rate up with certain workouts. I just love that. Because so many kettlebell workouts are ballistic in nature (meaning not just isometric movement with up and down reps) they can quickly rev up your heart rate. You can also improve flexibility and mobility in general with these types of workouts, which leads me into our next topic.

Flexibility and Mobility

This is the part that most people ignore. No one has time for that, right? It's all about burning those calories. Think again. Flexibility and mobility are so extremely important for so many reasons. What most people don't realize is that when you leave this part out, you are actually limiting your ability to gain more strength and move better in your workouts, therefore achieving greater results. Without full range of motion, exercises like squats, for example, cannot be performed as well. You may require better hip mobility, or sometimes it may be a lack of calf mobility that is not allowing you to get low enough in your squat. Or if you are lacking shoulder mobility, overhead movements may not be done as well as they could be. These types of situations can go on and on. You are also increasing your risk of injury when this is ignored.

Let's see how great your results will be when you can't even workout at all because of an injury that could have been avoided had you properly prepared your body with some mobility work to better perform your workout. Taking enough time to warm up effectively and also cool down and stretch after a workout is absolutely necessary. Not only this, but I advocate for taking days when this is ALL you work on. It's that important. I don't know about you, but I definitely want to move well long into my old age. I don't want to be someone who can't bend over to tie my own shoes or require assistance doing everyday things that I would otherwise be able to do on my own if I had proper mobility.

As nurses, we've seen it all. We've seen all kinds of patients who can hardly do anything for themselves when, honestly, it's not necessary. I don't want that to be me. I want to keep my joints and muscles freely moving to do all my own activities of daily living all by myself. It is certainly possible. And I know that means starting now, not when I'm old. As nurses, we really need to take some hints from our patients we see on a daily basis. This should be driving us even harder to do the things we know we need to do.

Yoga is such an incredible workout for so many reasons, but the most important in my mind is the benefit of good mobility.   I prefer yoga over static stretching by far. When you can move in flowing motion that is patterned in a way to provide great mobility to all of your joints and muscles it is much safer (and enjoyable in my mind) than just holding a static stretch. When people only use static stretching (especially on cold muscles that aren't even warmed up yet) they can actually do more damage than good.

More often than not, many people tend to push too far into a stretch, thus causing injury to a muscle rather than helping it. This can cause micro tearing of muscles and connective tissue. When we stretch too far, or too long this can cause the fascial tissue to lose the ability to recoil and the connective tissue can lose its elasticity, ultimately becoming less functional. This is the opposite of what we're trying to do, so be careful! For this reason, I feel that yoga is such a great way to gain these benefits.

You may not be loose at the beginning of a yoga session, and that's okay. You may not move as well at first getting in and out of certain movements. Be patient. The more times you go through a certain flow of movements, you will notice your body responding and becoming more pliable each time as your muscles get warmer. This is a safe way to get the best results. Once you are warm, then by all means some static stretching can be great, as long as it's done properly and never pushed to the point of pain. Always listen to your body and take certain cues it may be giving you. If something doesn't feel good, don't do it. There is no shame in not doing a certain pose or movement that does not feel right to your body.

And please realize that we are all different here. You may be naturally tighter in certain areas while others can reach amazing levels of flexibility with minimal effort in that same position that seems so far out of your reach. Some can make it look so easy to stretch deeply and get into all kinds of funky poses that maybe you or I will never achieve. That's okay. Be okay with that. Let it go.

I, personally, am not very flexible. This is honestly one of the reasons I became a sport yoga instructor. If you want to get good at something, teach it, right? That being said, I am still not the most flexible person, but I certainly have improved over time. You can't expect that after a few yoga sessions and then only doing it once in a great while that you are going to maintain great flexibility and mobility just from that. It really should be practiced regularly. I actually hated yoga the first couple of times I tried it. I found it awkward, uncomfortable, and I really just didn't understand it. I also have a hard time sitting still, so I felt like I was wasting valuable time. I was all about quick movements and I wanted to feel like I was super productive with any time I was devoting to exercise. Little did I know, I WAS being productive, I was just too stubborn and blind to see it at first.

> "The nature of yoga is to shine the light of awareness into the darkest corners of the body."
> -Jason Crandell

Then one day it hit me. I remembered just how amazing I felt AFTER the class was done. That was it. That feeling was great, and I wanted more of that. My body felt so loose, so relaxed, and I had such a sense of calm. It was awesome. I may not have loved everything we did during the class, but that after feeling was just the best thing ever. I slept better. My soreness from my hard workouts diminished more quickly. I felt good. I needed that again. And so began my love for yoga. Now I actually DO enjoy what is done during a class or a session that I may do on my own. I have learned to customize my yoga practice to do things in a way that is enjoyable for me so I will want to do it again. And now it is a gift to me.

Aside from better flexibility and mobility, yoga can provide great stress relief and an overall sense of well-being when practiced regularly. With breathing exercises done in yoga, a greater sense of mindfulness can be achieved as well. Calm your mind, relax your body and benefit from the relaxing sense of better well-being. These are all positive effects that all nurses (and anyone in general) can certainly benefit from as part of an exercise plan. When yoga is practiced on a regular basis, you can train yourself to be a more calm person in general. It can better equip you to handle those out of control situations that come up in everyday life. This goes way beyond just what's done on the yoga mat. Let it carry over into your life outside.

Practicing yoga and mindfulness in general can also help you in making better decisions for your health in other areas as well. I have read studies saying that people who practice yoga are more likely to make better food choices than those who do not. Why is this? I seriously believe it is because of that overwhelming sense of well-being that is achieved during yoga. You feel like you just did something so good and beneficial to your body, and you don't want to ruin that. It makes it pretty hard to go straight to a McDonald's drive through and order a Big Mac with a side of fries directly after a good yoga class. It's just not that likely. Although it is interesting to notice how many people, on the other hand, feel like they have "earned" their right to pig out after some other kind of hard workout session. Sure, you may be hungry and need to refuel after a difficult workout, but by no means does this give you a free pass to stuff your face on junk. Side note, end of discussion.

All this to say, if you have never tried yoga, I would highly recommend giving it a chance. You just might find that you love it, and it could possibly even become your favorite part of exercise in general. You don't know until you try! And what a gift for nurses. I truly think that if all nurses practiced some kind of yoga on a weekly basis, their overall health could certainly improve, possibly even making a very large impact on their life as a whole.

Throw out the Word Exercise

After all that discussion on different modes of exercise, let's be real. Some of us hate that word. It makes us cringe. Some of us may have to actually throw that word right out of our vocabulary, and that's okay. The word exercise carries a lot of baggage and negative connotation for many people. Many of us have spent years thinking of all exercise as punishment for being bad, or something you have to do because you're not good enough the way you are. We're called lazy if we don't do it and get grief from others if we're slacking. We have to sweat and be miserable doing this "exercise" because we're told to. Well then just forget it. What if there was something else we could do? Another way to look at it?

Kids play. They play for hours and hours at a time, and that is their exercise. What if adults did more play? Why not? What if we ran around the yard with our kids, tackling them in a pile of leaves? What if we played soccer in the yard, or chased the dog around with a toy? That's activity, and it's fun. Maybe that's what you need to focus on right now instead of planned exercise.

What if we just thought of movement in general? How our bodies move and work is actually quite amazing, isn't it? Even the simple act of going for a long walk, crawling on the ground after your toddler, dancing at a wedding (or in your living room!), throwing a ball, pulling your kids on a sled. Just move, do it often, and enjoy that in itself. Have you ever copied a toddlers movements? Man, they have squatting down to perfection! Squatting, crawling, jumping up off the ground.... that's a workout right there just moving like a toddler! They're not "exercising", they're living and moving.

How about just exploring? Going on a long hike and find something new. Explore a new bike path to see what birds or other wild life you might see. Go kayaking or paddle boarding and enjoy a new view. Climb a mountain with some friends.

Instead of exercise, how about training for something specific? Maybe you have a goal to become a black belt in karate. Or maybe you've always wanted to do one of those crazy adventure races with your friends. So you train to reach that specific goal because it has meaning to you. You're getting great exercise, without using that word. You're training with a purpose. Train hard, reach your goal and be proud of that!

Long story short, just move. Enjoy life. Get out and do things. Don't "exercise" with that old mentality if that has burned you in the past. Change the way you look at it if you need to, and find joy in it. Make it exciting, a new adventure, and a new part of your daily plan. Enjoy it!

Take Care of Your Feet

Most people don't spend much time thinking about their feet when it comes to fitness. Do you realize that each one of your feet has 26 bones, 33 joints and over 100 muscles? If we don't have proper strength in our feet, this can eventually cause problems in your hips, spine, and even become a problem for your entire body. So often we shove our feet into restrictive footwear, thus causing issues with the way our feet move and respond to movement. We spend long hours on our feet (especially as nurses), and often neglect the need to care for them with proper stretching and strengthening. Plantar fasciitis can be a nagging problem that comes up when our feet are not strong enough and stretched properly. Doing exercises to strengthen and mobilize your feet along with your calf muscles can do wonders for treating and preventing this issue. Our feet give us our foundation. They provide us with valuable information about the surface we are walking on. I especially like to be barefoot when weight training (particularly with squats and dead lifts). This helps greatly with stability and grounding yourself to better feel the surface you are working against. Doing balancing yoga poses with bare feet is great for this as well. Go barefoot sometimes, and be good to your feet!

Chapter Six

Stress and the Nurse

The word stress almost goes hand in hand with the profession of nursing. It is certainly not an easy job that you can take lightly, that's for sure. This is clear when you actually look at how many individuals enter the field of nursing to either drop out of nursing school before they finish, or find out in their first nursing job that the stress is too much for them to handle, and end up leaving the profession altogether. By no means am I putting any blame here either. This is understandable. Although some nursing jobs are clearly more stressful than others, a nurse is always responsible for the safety of another human's life. That alone, holds an awful lot of weight.

Of course it is true that many nurses seem to thrive on the stress and adrenaline of the job, and that is all well and good. There is a certain satisfaction that is reached when we make it through extremely tense and stressful situations involving saving someone's life, no doubt. That can be very rewarding. Yet, on the other hand, some of those extremely stressful times do not always end well. Nor do they go smoothly. This can leave a nurse feeling defeated, exhausted, empty and drained. Too much of this kind of stress ends up taking a toll on the nurse who may have once thrived in this type of atmosphere. It creeps up on us and we may not even realize it's happening. We may not see the effects this chronic stress is having on our own health. It becomes the daily grind. We try to just get used to it. Meanwhile, it can eat us up, steal our peace and take our own health right down the drain. Burnout is the next step. This is the dangerous spiral that needs to be stopped before it is too late.

Think of the most stressful nursing shift you've ever had. What was that like? Maybe you've had many different nursing jobs and had many different kinds of stresses along the way. This is a reality for many. Jobs like emergency nursing, critical care nursing, and med-flight nursing can certainly be very high stress dealing with life and death situations on a daily basis. You have to be ready to deal with anything coming through the door at any minute as an ER nurse. In a critical care setting, you are keeping alive the sickest of the sickest patients, sometimes managing multiple high-tech machines, and all the while caring for the patient themselves. Med-flight nurses are transporting patients who are in extreme situations and needing immediate care.

I spent most of my career in critical care and that's what I was most used to. But wow, was I in for a rude awakening when I had to float to a med-surg floor or an orthopedic floor. That's a whole different kind of stress! Sure, the patients may not be as critical, but now you're juggling multiple patients and dealing with the stress of keeping everything straight and getting all your work done before the end of your shift. You're answering multiple call lights and dealing with all sorts of issues because these patients can talk!

Then there's maternity nursing. The thought of a baby flying out at me when the doctor is not yet in the room absolutely horrifies me. I give those nurses credit. Not to mention, it sounds like a happy job, but when it's sad, it's really sad. And pediatrics? OUCH! Sick children. That takes a special breed. Not only are you taking care of that sick child, but now you have the added stress of caring for the stressed out, worried sick parents of that sick child. I cannot even imagine.

Oncology nurses. You are hard core. What a tough patient population to encounter on a daily basis. Home care nurses. You are the eyes for that patient. No one else is monitoring them in their home. It's up to you to make sure you're not missing anything and that you are communicating everything as effectively as possible in your charting. And the list goes on. I know I am leaving some out, but you get the gist of what I'm saying here. Every type of nursing has its own stresses.

Sometimes it's not the type of nursing job that is the source of the most stress. Sometimes it's people. Yes. You know it, and I know it. We've all worked with people in the medical field who are not all that easy to deal with. Can you say surgeon? Yeah, some of them don't exactly have a reputation for being nice. Of course there are exceptions and I can think of quite a few! But we have all heard stories of some surgeon having a power trip with a nurse. Surgeons need to be precise. They can't afford mistakes. This causes them to have a desire for perfection in all things related to their patients. But when things aren't "perfect", the blame has to go somewhere, and it very often goes straight to the nurse. Sometimes, it's all your fault no matter what you did or didn't do. The blame has to go somewhere, and you're an easy target. If you did do something, well then of course you shouldn't have. If you didn't do that same thing, then of course you should have. You can't win. There is no right answer.

I used to take this stuff personally, until I learned better. It is what it is (like I said, of course there are exceptions). But when a nurse is trying their hardest to care for a sick patient the best they know how, and all their efforts are shot down with a few blows from a hot-tempered doctor, that causes a lot of unnecessary pressure on the nurse. This creates a much more stressful atmosphere than anyone wants or needs.

And let's not forget having a stressful code situation go even worse with some angry doctor yelling in the room to escalate the drama and chaos. Not nice, and certainly very stressful. Ever get that tightness in your shoulders and bottom of your neck from those tense situations? I have. Ever wonder what your own blood pressure is at those times? This makes me appreciate so much more when things actually go smoothly in those situations, because the potential for utter chaos is always there.

Let me be clear, I am not bashing doctors here. I have had the privilege of working with many amazing doctors who are incredible human beings. Many of them have such a huge respect for the nurses caring for their patients, and this can make all the difference in a working relationship. It is, however, unfortunate when some doctor/nurse relationships are not as smooth as we would like.

And I hate to say it, but of course it's not just doctors that cause the stress. There are certainly other nurses that can make a situation unbearable for us. We all know there are difficult people in every job. Every profession in life has its own group of peers that cause unnecessary stress. It's just life, and we know that. We've all heard that nurses eat their young, right? I've seen that before and I'm sure you have too if you've been a nurse for a while. Or worse, maybe it happened to you.

This chapter might make it sound like nursing is a horrible career. That is NOT where I'm going with this, please understand. We all became nurses for a reason, and there is plenty to love about the profession. I am simply bringing to light the stresses that us nurses deal with continually, and sometimes don't even realize the effects these have on our own health. I am certainly not suggesting you quit your job (or maybe you need to if it's THAT bad), but recognizing the stress as an issue is the first step in trying to do something about it.

We can't change the fact that patients are going to code. We can't change the personalities of those around us. We can't change the entire nature of our job description depending on what type of nursing we do. So what's there to do? Help the nurse take care of the nurse.

If every nurse had appropriate sources of stress relief for themselves, this can be such a huge benefit to their health while maintaining a nursing career that they enjoy. Don't let the stress of your career ruin you. Recognize when it is too much, and maybe some adjustments do need to be made. Maybe it truly is time for a job change. Maybe you just need to cut down your hours a little bit each week (if financially possible). Maybe YOU are actually the cause of a lot of the stress in your job! Yeah, I said it. If you are the one stirring up the chaos, adding to the drama, escalating stressful situations, and making life hard on others, then maybe, just maybe you can adjust some actions yourself. You will actually be doing yourself a huge favor along with your colleagues. Be the kind of nurse you want to work with. Imagine if we all did that? It wouldn't be so bad!

Let's examine the meaning of stress first. First of all, stress in general isn't bad for us. We need some types of stress every day. It keeps us motivated to be able to adapt to our surroundings at any given time. This is a positive influence on our lives. The problem comes when we have too much stress that is beyond what we perceive as possible for us to handle. We judge this in our minds by asking ourselves how important the current situation is to us specifically, and do we really have the resources to cope with this situation?

This is a huge reason as to why some nurses deal with stressful situations much better than others. Stress is not an entity of its own, and different people will perceive the same stressor in a different light. Stress is the response our mind and body has based on the perceived tension or threat of a situation. Stress is not what happens to you. It's what you THINK happens to you. I used to have a hard time with this as a young nurse. Sometimes it's difficult to quiet your mind and truly think of how bad a situation really is, and is it truly necessary to let yourself get all stressed out about it? It can often be managed more easily than we think.

> "Stress is a function not of events, but of our view of those events."
> -Ellen Langer

Have you ever been in awe of a nurse who would be in the middle of a code seeming to be as cool as a cucumber, letting nothing faze them whatsoever as they continue along doing what needs to be done? That's a great attribute to have, and it's one that doesn't always come easy. But aside from a code situation, think of other stressful shifts in general. I remember being on orientation for my first nursing job in a surgical ICU setting. I had two patients. One of them was circling the drain, and the other was trying to leap out of bed with multiple tubes and lines attached to him. I didn't know what to pay attention to first. I was consumed with stress and felt like this was the worst day of my life. At that moment, my preceptor grabbed me by the shoulders. She looked me in the eye and said "This will end. It's twelve hours of your life, and it will be over soon. Gather your thoughts, prioritize, and let's do the best we can for the patients".

Those words stuck with me for a long time, and I still think of them from time to time. Because no matter how bad a shift is, it WILL end. All you can do is just focus on the next step and keep going to do the best you can for your patients. Don't let the stress of a situation ruin you to the point of you being no use to anyone. The situation will end, no matter what the outcome. It's temporary. Just clear your mind and focus on what needs to be done. Our own perception of things around us can either make or break our day.

What happens to us when we let stress get the best of us? There are certainly negative effects on our own health when we live in a chronic stressful state. Our immune system is less able to respond to invaders like a bacteria or virus. Our blood pressure rises. Our body secretes cortisol which increases fat storage (predominantly abdominal fat which can increase our risk of heart disease, diabetes and premature death). Our muscles tense up. Our sleep is disturbed. We tend to overeat (and it's usually not with healthy food). Some may resort to alcohol. It can be an ugly downward spiral if we don't grab hold of it before too long.

Managing Stress

There is help. There are definitely things we can do to combat this. Start first by recognizing that we need better control of the situation. Start becoming more mindful of when things begin to unravel inside. This is huge, and may take some practice. We may need to actually reduce the amount of stress if it is too much for us to handle.

Sometimes this just means saying no. Are you the one everyone always comes to when they need help because they know you'll never turn them down? Learn your limits. Know what the breaking point is for you, and draw that line. It's okay to say no. You'll live, and so will the person who wants something from you. In the name of saving your own sanity, the word "no" is a life saver. Get to know it. It can be hard for the giving, caretaker type that us nurses generally are. Trust me, you will be so glad when you learn how and when to appropriately say no to people. Weigh the situation in your mind, and see what's at stake. Are you already stretched super thin? Can you handle adding one more thing? Or is that your breaking point? Recognize it, give and help when you can, but know when you cannot. And that's okay. Perfectly okay. This is taking care of yourself, which is what this whole book is about. Start saying yes to saying no. You matter too.

How about avoiding arguments when possible? That's huge. If any of you work with toxic coworkers who constantly find reason to complain, argue and cause strife, steer clear. The only way to win with a toxic person is don't play the game. Don't even engage in the conversation. Minimize exposure to this as much as possible and go along your way. Engaging in it only eggs them on, and increases your stress. You don't need that, and they don't need the encouragement to keep on doing what they're doing. Leave it be.

My favorite way to squash stress in its tracks is to put things in perspective for a moment. If we can calm ourselves enough to just take a second and look at how the current situation may affect your entire rest of your life, it's usually very eye opening. Starting a gratitude journal can help here. When we focus on what we are truly grateful for, the stresses that frustrate us on any given day don't really hold as much weight anymore. Is your long ride to work in rush hour traffic really going to take away from the fact that you are truly grateful for the loving family you have at home? No. It has nothing to do with that and it can't ruin that gift.

Most of us are lucky enough to have a roof over our heads, clothes on our backs, and food to eat. That might seem expected to you, but realize that you are considered rich compared to the majority of the people in this world. Most of us have so much more than so many people all over the world. A stressful day at work can't take that from you. You're still blessed. Stressful moments can only hurt you as much as you allow them to. Don't give them that power. Don't let the stressful moments steal your joy of the good stuff and blind you from your blessings. I like to think of eternity here. Our lives on this earth are but a blink of an eye compared to eternity. How much can a stressful situation really hurt me? I know I will get through whatever is upon me, and you will too. Stress isn't coming with me when I go. It does no good to me here on this earth for the time I'm here, and it has no weight on my eternity whatsoever. More on this in another chapter coming up, but for now, just put stress in a little temporary box and push it to the side because it doesn't matter in the end.

"Taking good care of you means the people in your life will receive the best of you rather than what's left of you."
-Carl Bryan

A little mindful meditation can go a long way as well. It's hard to make ourselves sit still sometimes, right? Sure. I know it has been an issue for me at times. There's always something that needs to be done, so how can I possibly justify sitting still? And by myself? It just seems wrong when we have so many things on our to-do list and other people to take care of. There's that nurturer again.

We can't fathom an actual moment to ourselves without feeling guilty. Isn't that wrong of me to expect that? It seems selfish and just not possible. This is what we need to let go. It most certainly IS okay and completely necessary for us to sit from time to time in a moments peace and be alone. You need that. We all need that. And it is perfectly acceptable. Not only do we need to do this, but we need to make it a priority! Yes! You actually need to come first sometime, because if you don't, you will eventually be no good to anyone around you.

Sit. Take time to hear yourself breathe. Get in a comfortable position, and just be. Empty your mind of any and all things that need to be done in your busy day. Notice your breathing in and out. Feel the air entering and filling your lungs. You may even want to hold your breath in for a count of three, then slowly release the air, noticing your lungs deflating. Try to completely relax all the muscles in your body and let go of any tension you notice. Do this for at least a full five to ten minutes. This can create a sense of mindfulness that can help bring so much peace and clarity back into our day, and ultimately help us to better manage our stress. Complete silence is great for this, I think, but if you need a little quiet music in the background to help you, that's fine too. Just don't let the music distract you. There are even apps you can get on your phone for meditation and breathing exercises. Check them out!

Yoga, as mentioned earlier in this book, is a super stress reliever. When you can combine purposeful breathing with movement that helps release tension, that is a beautiful thing. The more often you practice yoga, the greater results you will see carry over into your everyday life, especially with managing stress.

Magnesium is something that so many of us are deficient in and don't realize it. Both emotional and physical stress can be a cause of magnesium deficiency. Stress depletes magnesium stores in our body, and when we replace this, our stress can be somewhat relieved. Our muscles need a proper magnesium/calcium balance to be able to relax. Replacing necessary magnesium can help decrease nervousness, irritability and help us to better relax overall. It is the anti-stress mineral! I like to use powdered forms and mix them in liquid because it is better absorbed this way rather than a pill. I highly recommend checking this out if you have a lot of stress in your life and have never addressed a possibly magnesium deficiency. It could be a life saver. However, this should not be a replacement for addressing other ways to control your stress as needed. Don't ignore the other stuff and think you can fix it all with magnesium.

You can find more information about this on my website nursegonestrong.com. There are other natural substances you can look into as well for stress, but as always, first address where you can cut back on the stressors in the first place before just looking for a quick fix. And be sure to always ask your doctor first if adding a supplement is right for you before starting anything new.

As mentioned earlier in this book, it's no secret at this point that exercise can also greatly help relieve symptoms of stress. This is huge, and such an obvious one in my life. Nothing rids my day of stress better than a good workout. It's just so true. I feel ten times better afterwards, and I am usually able to look at a stressful situation from a different angle when I am done. Exercise has this way of washing our minds and getting the junk out, leaving a much clearer view of what is and is not important. That's a gift, and it's free. There's no pill needed. Exercise is so underused and under-prescribed for this reason. So many people are so quick to take a pill before resorting to some enjoyable physical activity that only has GOOD side effects. Do this first.

How does eating right help with stress? More than you know! Most of us reach for the comfort food in times of stress, right? Just making things even worse. And talk about feeding the fire when you're having a stressful day at work and then you walk past the nurse's station. What do you see? So often there is candy or other high sugar treats laying around that someone brought in to make the nurses "happy". That's all well meaning and good at times, but it just sets you up for such a trap when we fall into that mentality that it's there to help us. After that initial sugar rush, these foods actually leave us feeling lethargic, unclear in our thinking and not really motivated to do much of anything. Avoid it if you can!

Healthy high fiber carbohydrate food can give your that little boost of serotonin that makes us feel good, yet doesn't give us that nasty crash. Try veggies over rice, sweet potatoes, or some sweet fruit. Not that you are going to find any of this at the nurse's station (ha-ha), but in general these types of foods can give us the comfort feeling we need, yet also leave us with some energy in the tank. How about caffeine? Now I love my coffee, and I know there are plenty of you out there too. Just be mindful when too much might be too much. If your coffee intake is leaving you jittery all the time with an unsettled feeling like you are unable to relax, then it may be time to dial it back a bit. Pay attention to your sleep as well. Is your coffee intake (either amount or timing) affecting your sleep? This is not going to help reduce stress in your life if your caffeine intake is disturbing you from getting enough sleep. Just be mindful.

What are your sleep habits in general? Could that area use some help? Any night shift nurses out there? Ouch. Talk about a nightmare of trying to get enough sleep and feel normal on any given day when your flipping back and forth from daytime sleep to nighttime sleep. I worked nights myself for ten years, and I know the struggle very well. I also realize that there are many of you out there who (by some miracle of God) are able to sleep great despite your night shift routine. More power to you! It can be a challenge for many, that's for sure. Make sure to optimize your environment the best you possibly can if you need to sleep during the day and flip back and forth from day/night sleeping. Do your best... I know it's a challenge!

The importance of sleep is often underrated. Most adult need between 7-9 hours of sleep per night, yet many don't come close. Lacking sleep will certainly not help your stress levels go down one bit, and it will most likely add to more issues. Many studies have been done showing the benefits of getting enough sleep in relation to overall health. Long term effects of not getting enough sleep can lead to weight gain, high blood pressure, depression, higher risk for diabetes and some cancers, and also premature aging. Yuck. Nothing good there. Most of us love our sleep, yet fail to make it a priority. We have too much to do, yet once again. It's time to make time for sleep. Our bodies deserve that time to rest, recover, unwind, and recharge to face the next day (or night, if you are a night shifter!). And if you're trying to jump on the exercise band wagon, it is imperative that you get enough sleep to perform a good workout, and also recover from it. Your muscles need that, and your entire body will thank you.

So how does lacking sleep add to weight gain? One main reason is the relation of a couple of hormones called leptin and ghrelin. These two hormones have a lot to do with our hunger signals and appetite control. Leptin is secreted mostly by fat cells, and it decreases our hunger. Ghrelin, on the other hand, is secreted from the stomach and signals us to feel hungry. You might think then that the more fat you have, the more leptin you secrete and should not feel hungry, right? Not really, since you can actually become leptin resistant with obesity, but that's another story. A lack of sleep actually causes a decrease in leptin levels (therefore not getting that satisfied feeling that we should from normal levels) and causes and increase in ghrelin (causing us to feel even more hungry than normal). Not cool, right? I know I have noticed that myself for sure. Think of times you've been severely lacking sleep. Did you just want to keep eating all the time? I know I have. Get your sleep so you can keep these hormones in check, along with avoiding all the other pitfalls that come along with sleep deprivation.

Something I use in my own home to help with sleep and stress relief is essential oils (lavender especially). I have an essential oil diffuser and I love to use this often. I find that the lavender oil promotes such a calming effect on my mind and body, and it truly helps me fall off to sleep much better. You might want to give this a try! There are many other great oils with other benefits that I love as well. You can find these on my website at nursgonestrong.com.

10 Tips for Better Sleep

-Try to wake up and go to bed at the same time each day (I know, hard for night-shifters!).

-Exercise, but not within 2 hours of bedtime (if possible).

-Avoid electronics or television within 1-2 hours of bed.

-Wind down with a book, meditation, or relaxation breathing before bed (this can be as short as 5-10 minutes and be beneficial).

-Avoid drinking alcohol before bed, or avoid it altogether. Although alcohol may help you to fall asleep, it can cause you to wake up during your sleep.

-See if a magnesium supplement can help, like Natural Calm, or try 1-2 teaspoons of raw honey before bed.

-Create a calming atmosphere in your bedroom. Use a Himalayan salt lamp and/or diffuse some lavender essential oil before bed.

-Try some yoga poses or light stretches before bedtime.

-Take caution with any sleeping pills. They should be for short term solutions only, not something you rely on every night.

-Journal before bed. Many people have trouble sleeping because they go to bed worrying about too many things. Journaling about what you are grateful for and also even getting some worries out on paper can help you relax your mind before bed and get to sleep with less worry.

Chapter Seven

Decreasing Toxins

I want to live a healthy life, and I want to encourage others to do the same. I think that is clear at this point, right? Well this next topic doesn't exactly come to mind for most people when we talk about living a healthy life. Everyone focuses on the two biggies - diet and exercise. While I would agree that those probably are the two most important factors in this equation, it's not all there is. As we saw in the last chapter, certainly stress can have a major impact on one's health and wellness. But what about toxins? Honestly, they're all around us just waiting to wreak havoc on our body. Thankfully we have a liver which does a great job at filtering so much out for us, but I want to make sure I'm not adding more toxic junk than my body can handle to the point where it's causing disease.

If we are going to try so hard being healthy in all these other ways, we need to look at how toxins can affect us. So what's the big deal? When our bodies are bombarded with too many toxins, they can cause damage to cell mitochondria (the power house of the cell), cause a decrease in thyroid hormones, and some can even decrease the ability of our bodies to burn fat. That's not cool! First, let's look at what toxins are sneaking in right on our produce that we are ingesting more of lately so we can be healthy.

Pesticides are a huge source of toxins that many of us ingest daily. Some fruits can even have thirty or more different pesticides applied during their growth. That's a lot! Did you know you were eating all that right along with your yummy apple? Probably not. And apples are my favorite! An apple a day keeps the doctor away, right? That's all well and good until we look at what's been sprayed all over that apple. Here is the danger. Pesticides have been linked to many different cancers, Alzheimer's disease, Parkinson's disease, autism, attention deficit hyperactivity disorder, and several birth defects.

These are many of the things we're trying to avoid with our healthy eating and exercise, yet all this junk is on so many of our healthy food choices themselves. Not good. So what choice do we have? Yes, we can buy organic fruits and vegetables when possible. Organic farmers do still use pesticides themselves, yet they use much less than conventional farmers and they use more natural sources. They do not use synthetic pesticides, and organic farmers are strictly regulated to hold to these standards. The choices they use are more friendly to the environment, and ultimately more friendly to you. Organic produce can certainly be more expensive, and it may not always be available depending on where you live. The key here is to do the best you can.

Try to eat organic produce as much as possible for the foods that have the most pesticide use: things like apples, strawberries, blueberries, celery, tomatoes, spinach, grapes, cucumbers, peaches, bell peppers and nectarines. You can look up the "dirty dozen" list to see what produce has used the most pesticides for each year and try to always buy organic off that list whenever possible. You can also look up the "clean fifteen" list to see what produce usually uses the least amount of pesticides, making them safe choices to buy conventionally grown. Don't make yourself crazy here by any means. Just do the best with the choices you have available to you, and always know that eating your fruits and vegetables should never be avoided because you can't find them all organic. The benefit of eating these foods outweighs the risk of NOT eating any of them because you're trying to avoid pesticides.

> "Your diet is a bank account. Good food choices are good investments."
> -Bethenny Frankel

Do you ever think of the pesticides that could be in your own home? Many of us have conventional insect sprays and weed killers that we use around ourselves and our family members all the time. Breathing that stuff in is so dangerous. There are warnings all over those labels, yet we continue to use them to get the job done. There are other options. Just look up toxic free ways to kill insects or weeds on your lawn. There is a ton of information and tons of options out there. Go for the cleaner options for the sake of your health!

Health and beauty products are another source of toxins that many of us don't realize. Almost one third of all personal care products out there contain one or more ingredients that are classified as possible human carcinogens. What we spray on our hair and rub on our skin every day soaks right in through our pores. Do you ever pay attention to ingredients in things like body lotion, face creams, shampoo, deodorant or even toothpaste? I don't want possible carcinogens leaking into my body when I'm trying to live a healthy lifestyle and avoid this stuff. It's no joke.

The USDA claims that the small amount that are in these products are safe. But who's regulating how much of how many different products people are using on a daily basis? Who's keeping track of all the many different harmful ingredients getting into your skin every day? It's impossible to gauge the true risk. The USDA has no idea how many different toxins you, specifically, are exposed to on a daily basis with multiple different products. I would rather avoid as many as possible just to be safe.

Parabens are one of those harmful ingredients that we find in so many beauty products. These have been found in breast cancer tissue. How about triclosan? That's the ingredient found in so many antibacterial soaps and some toothpastes. It has been linked to cancer. Dyes and fragrances that are added to so many lotions can disrupt your endocrine system and mess with your hormones. Aluminum is found in so many antiperspirant/deodorants. It has been linked to breast cancer, Alzheimer's disease and kidney problems. Whether they can prove that these claims are all absolutely true or not, the fact that it is in question and some studies have shown links to this is enough for me to avoid these ingredients. I'm certainly not doing myself any harm by trying to find safer options out there, so that is what I choose. A great resource for checking the safety of certain beauty products is www.cosmeticsdatabase.com. See how your favorite products rate! I make my own deodorant at home using coconut oil, baking soda and essential oils. It's all natural, completely safe, it works, and it's really not that hard!

Homemade Deodorant

-1/4 cup coconut oil (slightly softened but not liquid)

-2 Tablespoons baking powder

-1 Tablespoon arrowroot powder

-15 drops of lavender essential oil (find my favorite on my website at nursegonestrong.com)

Mix all ingredients until smooth and keep in a small mason jar. Coconut oil will become liquid above 76 degrees Fahrenheit , but just stir before use and it will be fine.

Do you know what's in your cleaning products? This is one thing that really kind of bothers me at work. The harsh smell of so many cleaning products used in the hospital is really tough to take sometimes. I have zero control over that, and I understand that. But I do have control over what I choose to use in my own house. Many of the same harmful chemicals that are in health and beauty products are also found in cleaning products, and then some!

Do you know that using vinegar and baking soda is a very effective way to clean many surfaces in your home? I actually love sprinkling baking soda on bathroom surfaces and then spraying white vinegar from a spray bottle over the baking soda. It bubbles up and foams instantly, so this may satisfy some of you visual people who need to SEE it working! Try it. Again, look up options for toxin free cleaning for your home. There are tons of options out there. You don't have to make your own either. There are good products out there that use plant based ingredients and they clean very well. Mrs. Meyer's and Method cleaning products are great non-toxic cleaners that I have been very happy with myself. Give them a shot!

Make sure you are always drinking plenty of water also to help your body rid itself of any and all toxins that we do come in contact with. This is important obviously for health in general, but don't forget that your helping the detoxification process in your body as well when you make sure to drink enough water every day. Flush it out!

Chapter Eight

Self Doubt, Fear and Body Image

Doubt. It's a tough little beast to get a handle on sometimes, isn't it? It attacks the best of us, and some more often than others. It's that nasty, snarky, sneaky voice inside of us that lies to us. It fills us with complete garbage, and we actually believe it way more often than we should. The body believes what the mind says. Doubt holds you back from the life you are meant to enjoy. It can riddle us with fear, and paralyze us from making any positive moves that we know may actually benefit us in the long run. This robs us out of living life to the fullest! This takes your possible successes and throws them to the side like garbage. When we doubt our ability to do something, it makes starting and finishing any task

> "Whether you think you can or you think you can't, you're right."
> -Henry Ford

so much more work than it ever needed to be than if we just didn't doubt in the first place.

So what do we get out of doubt? If it has such a strong hold on us, what purpose does it serve? None. We get nothing. We get robbed from all the good stuff that we actually could have done in our life. When doubt holds you back, you ultimately lose. We sit on the sidelines of life and let everyone else go on by achieving their goals and dreams while we sit there next to that ugly doubt that stole our future. We doubt that we can ever eat right, or lose weight, or stick to something we need to do. We doubt our abilities at work, our worth in helping others, and even our basic contribution to society sometimes. Don't believe the lie. Fear cripples us. It tells us it's too scary to actually TRY to achieve something or do something new.

What if I fail? What if I mess up? What if I get hurt? What if I can't do it? What if it's too hard? So what? Failure is a stepping stone to success. It is a necessary means by which to achieve great things. We all fail. We all stumble and skin a knee from time to time. But we get up, and try again when we say no to doubt and fear. Setbacks happen to anyone who ever takes a risk. Ask any successful person out there who is a master at what they do. Ask them if they ever failed. I guarantee the answer is yes. And probably more than once. Ask them if they sat back and listened to that little voice of doubt in their head before they went on and achieved their dreams. I bet not, because if they did, they wouldn't be where they are. They may have heard that voice at one time try to change their path, but they knew better than to follow that lead... at least in the end. Be stronger than that inner demon that does not have your best interest at heart. If we give in, we allow the ultimate self betrayal, because we are the ones stopping ourselves from the good stuff.

So how do we deal with this? First you need to recognize it for what it is, and acknowledge when it appears. Then say STOP. You need to stop doubt in its tracks and don't let it go on another step further into your brain. The more we dwell on it and the longer we allow it to hang around, the further away you get from living the life you were meant to live. Recognizing this is the first step. Get to know that feeling of when it shows up, and be aware of its presence.

Then we need to ask ourselves some questions. Ask yourself how many times in the past when you have doubted or feared situations, did that awful negative thing you imagined happening actually come to be? Most of the time, it's not very often that we can come up with such recollections. That is because our doubt and fear tend to magnify the worst possible case scenario every time, when in actuality, it's pretty unlikely to happen.

Next, recognize if there are common threads. Are you feeling doubt and fear with certain situations only when you are around specific people or specific events? Explore that, and write down when you notice yourself coming up with these thoughts. Get to the bottom of why that is, and attack it. You just might be missing out on something great. Not much comes from a life that never takes a risk. Most amazing experiences or dreams come true almost always involve some risk. Don't be afraid to cash in on that.

I will share a brief story of my own on this topic. Back in 2010 I was given the opportunity to go on a medical mission trip to Kenya. When I first heard of this chance, I was so excited and filled with enthusiasm for actually having the chance to do this. Going on a mission trip was something I always wanted to do. I had heard stories from friends of mine about such awesome experiences, and I had thought about it for years.

But then when it came time to actually sign up and put a deposit down on a plane ticket, fear set in, and it set in hard. I had young kids at the time. How could I leave them for 15 days and go to another continent? What if something happened to them while I was gone and I wasn't here? What if my plane crashed or I got killed over there somehow? What if this was IT! Then I also heard myself trying to talk myself out of the need for going anyway. Well it wasn't a good time, or I'm too old now for that, or I probably wouldn't really like it as much as I think I would. I wrestled with this for weeks, and it tore me up. I used up so much time, energy and thought on this doubt and fear.

Finally, I decided I had to go. I needed to take this risk for something I had always dreamed of doing. So I went. And to this day, that trip was one of the most life changing experiences I have ever had. The sights I saw, the people I was able to help and the amazing experience of just being in Kenya absolutely blew my mind. Seeing those people up close and personal with their illnesses, but also their joy... it was something I'll never forget.

I learned many life lessons on that trip, and also was able to sponsor a child from the orphanage we were at while we were there. Writing to him and receiving letters from him is always a highlight for my entire family. We now have a lifelong connection with someone that I otherwise never would have experienced had I not gone.

What if I never went? What if I gave in to fear and doubt? I would've missed out on all those blessings. All those experiences. All those life lessons and all the joy of so many beautiful people. Not only was I able to help others and experience that joy, but I was blessed myself in so many ways by the people I met and the experiences I was able to be a part of. And guess what? My kids were absolutely fine. Nothing happened to anyone while I was gone, and nor did my plane go down. I didn't get hurt or killed while I was gone, but rather I came back more whole than when I left. It was pure beauty. It changed me. It made me more me, and I loved that. Now I know that if an opportunity comes up that scares me a little bit, I know that it is probably something I need to do. :-)

Since that trip, I have made it a point to do something new every year that scares me. The following year in 2011, I did my first Tough Mudder race. The thought of running 13 miles up a mountain through mud, jumping into ice cold water, running through electrical wires, crawling in dark spaces and jumping off a platform that was way too high for my comfort zone did NOT sound appealing to me. It scared me. And at the same time, I wanted it bad. I wanted to face my fear and say I did it. And I did. That just sparked a love for adventure races and I have done many more since. Facing your fears is a powerful thing. It's exhilarating, freeing and opens up all kinds of possibilities.

So no matter what you fear or what you doubt, please take a moment and think about what it is possibly robbing you of. What is it taking from you that is rightfully yours and possibly at your fingertips? What are you passing up in the name of fear and doubt? Don't pass up all that good stuff. It's waiting for you; to change you, mold you, refine you and allow you to be who you truly are. Growth lies on the other side. That's where the meat is! Of course there is good reason to think about and carefully weigh decisions in life, but just make sure you know exactly what's holding you back. Life begins on the other side of fear. Don't let it win.

The Amazing Bill Bell

Bill never exercised as a kid. He never got to play sports or be very active. This carried on into his middle-aged years. Then at age 53, Bill had a stress test and the doctor was concerned that he may have some heart disease. He recommended Bill start jogging 2-3 days per week. Bill started to enjoy this, and after a few weeks he asked the doctor if he could run every day. His doctor agreed. One year later, Bill ran his first marathon, and went on to run 14 marathons that same year. At age 59 Bill signed up for swimming lessons to prepare for the swimming portion of an Ironman Triathlon, and two years later at age 61, he completed his first Ironman Triathlon competition (2.4 mile swim/112 mile bike/26.2 mile run). In his 60's and 70's, Bill went on to complete 32 Ironman races.

What can we take away from this? Sometimes you might just need a little nudge to get you going... and who knows how far you might go! This should be an inspiration to anyone out there who thinks they're too old to start exercising. Don't doubt yourself, and don't be afraid to know your limits!

Body Image

I am amazed at the number of women I have spoken to in the last several years who say that they struggle with this topic more than anything else (and this definitely seems to affect women much more than men). This topic is certainly not nurse specific of course, but I feel that it's important to bring up when discussing struggles with trying to live a healthy life, whether you are a nurse or not. How you view yourself can be a make it or break it issue in your life. It can control everything. Every move you make and every decision you weigh. It can consume every waking hour of your day if it is something you struggle with severely. However, it is quite often the case that your own perception of yourself is so far different from how others view you. But this is hard for us to see sometimes when we can't see past our own image problems.

Some girls can start worrying about their weight and body image as early as 6-7 years old. They don't want to get "fat". They don't want to be "ugly". This comes from many sources. Believe it or not, this can even stem from what seems to be such an innocent and fun thing for young girls - the Disney Princesses themselves. There aren't many "princesses" out there who aren't perfectly in shape with thin waste lines and perfect skin and hair. Every little girl dreams of being a princess. But what if they're not as pretty? What if they're not that thin? I am not blaming Disney here at all, and I think all those movies are great, but there is something crucial here that young kids need to understand. Those movies are a fantasy. Those animated characters are made in a fantasy world where everything is happily ever after and everyone looks perfect.

Kids need to know that as much as it's fun to dream and dress up like princesses, no one is requiring them to achieve that status in life. They are good enough, always, just as they are. They hear adults talking (so often their own parents) about being fat, or needing to be more thin... as if this is the only way they can be happy in life. This is something that can stay with these young girls long into their adult life. Be careful how you speak around your children (or any children) about body appearance and weight! This is crucial. They are listening to every word, and they are watching you. Our society has taught us for so long that there is only one accepted way to look. The supermodels we see on the covers of magazines are what we are to aim to look like, if we want to be anyone of any worth in life. This is an unrealistic expectation and standard of beauty that most of us will never achieve.

Teenage years can be painful for so many. It's all about your image when you're a teen, and body image issues continue to be on the rise. These years are filled with a rollercoaster of emotions and a strong desire to find our own identity. Who are we and what makes us important? Why do we matter at all? What worth, if any, do we have in this world? We struggle and wrestle with trying to fit in and be accepted, yet all the while wondering if we're ever good enough. The pressure to fit in is huge, and so many kids equate being thin and pretty enough as being the standard for achieving this.

> "No one can make you feel inferior without your consent."
> -Eleanor Roosevelt

The number one driver of the conditions known as anorexia and bulimia is body dissatisfaction. So many of us out there hate our physical bodies. Body Dysmorphic Disorder is a serious condition where a person develops an imagined defect in their appearance, and they can fixate on this defect or imagined flaw to the point where it becomes all consuming. This can require close watching and some intense counseling to heal. Some look in the mirror in disgust and shame. They see something so horrific that in no way resembles how others see them or who they truly are. That absolutely breaks my heart.

What about comparison? Who's played that game before? Isn't it so easy to go to the gym or out in a public place and immediately compare ourselves to others. We wish we looked like this one or that one. Why can't our arms, legs or abs look like that? How come I can't fit into that dress like she can? If we could only be that thin then our life would be great. Stop.

Comparison will cause an ugly cycle of negativity in your mind and it will take you nowhere good at all. We all have our own journey. We all have different bodies, and you may NEVER look like that person you keep comparing yourself to. It doesn't matter. You are you. You aren't them. Work on being the best version of YOU because the world needs that. The world doesn't need another version of someone else... it needs you. There is a reason for each one of us being on this earth, so don't waste that time trying to achieve someone else's status.

On the other hand, be careful if you are on the other end of the spectrum thinking that you HAVE achieved that standard and are now full of pride. Working hard for a healthy body and to be in good shape is all well and good, but don't tip over to the point of becoming prideful in your life because of it. This can have an ugly downfall of its own. Don't reward yourself because you think you have met the ideal standard the world gives. The world's standards should never be our judge of success anyway. And what good is having a body that measures up to the world's standards if you have an ugly prideful heart? Think about that. That's not success. That's a whole other problem in itself.

The best way to heal this nasty beast of the "ugly and never-good-enough" image of ourselves is to truly grasp the understanding that we are all made in the image of the one true and living God. He is where you get your worth. He is where you get your value. He made you and loves everything about you, even if you don't. God Himself, made you in His image, and you are here for a specific purpose. Our purpose ultimately is to reflect His image to the world. But instead, we focus on the world's image of who we think we should be. This is the biggest mistake we can make and can leave us spinning in this vicious cycle of never being enough.

The world's view will never satisfy us. We will always be struggling, reaching, trying and failing to achieve the perfect acceptance of the world. You are enough, just as you are. Let go of the struggle. Let go of the comparison. Let go of the anxiety and self loathing behavior. Be still and know that He is God (Psalm 46:10), and He made you and loves you just as you are. No strings attached. Be free in this acceptance and healing. Find your worth in Jesus Christ who made the ultimate sacrifice for you and me on the cross. That means you are worth so much more than any label the world might put on you.

Chapter Nine

The End of the Line

I am a huge advocate for taking care of one's self here on this earth. Our bodies truly are a gift, and we are only given one in this lifetime. I am all for treating it right and having it serve us well while we are here so we can enjoy life to the fullest. We have been entrusted with this amazing gift, and it is only right that we care for it the very best we can. However, we are all mortal. This body will not last us forever. No matter how much we exercise and eat right, it will die, for sure at some point.

As nurses, we see patients pass from this life all the time. Labor and delivery nurses get to see the beauty of life at the very beginning, and many other nurses in different settings see life in its last and final moments before passing on. The body can't fight any more after so long. This is always such an emotional and thought provoking time for a nurse. Some occasions hit us a little harder than others. We cry and we feel right along with the families very often. When a life here on earth is done, it just seems so final. But then what? What matters then?

If we try so hard while here on this earth to live life to the fullest and take the very best care of ourselves, wouldn't it make sense to care what happens for eternity after this body dies? I think so. Life passes like the blink of an eye, doesn't it? The older we get, the faster it seems to go. Even more reason to make the best of it while we're here! Compared to eternity, your life and mine is so small and insignificant. We won't spend very long here, in comparison. And where exactly are we going? Do you know? Have you ever thought of this while watching one of your patients pass on? Have you truly thought about your own eternity after your body dies? You will spend way more time in eternity than you will ever spend here on this earth. If you have never really thought about it, I encourage you to do so now.

Have you spent time with patients on their death bed? It is a heartbreaking time, for sure. But for some, it is also a time of great hope. When this mortal body starts to fail, there can be pain, suffering and exhaustion. It can be hard to watch. I love seeing family members gather around a patients bed to pray. When they truly know their loved one is going to a better place without any more pain and suffering, it can be a relief. It can be a time of hope and renewal as much as it is hard to see them go. But how do they know? How do they really know with such certainty that their loved one is going to spend eternity in a good place?

The Hope of Jesus Christ

I truly believe there is a way to know for sure. First of all, none of us are perfect, right? Absolutely not. We fail, we make mistakes, we hurt each other, we cheat, we lie, and the list goes on. We are not born "good". We are all born sinners. It's in our nature. Who taught a toddler how to have a temper tantrum? Or steal a toy right out of another child's hands? Or lie to their parents? Or disobey the rules? No one. We don't teach that to our kids. They (we) are all born with a sinful nature. We all have that instinctive "it's all about me" attitude inside of us somewhere. It's just who we are. Sure, we can be sorry and learn to do better as time goes on, but we will fail again. We will sin again. We are never going to be "sinless" and perfect in this life.

We are not inherently good, but we don't really like to admit this. At least we're not as bad as some other people. But the problem with this thinking is that the standard we are held to in order to enter heaven is not comparing us against some other human, it's comparing us to God and all His holiness. None of us fit the bill. Not one. Yet so many people think that because they are generally a "good" person, they certainly deserve to go to heaven. Why shouldn't they? It only makes sense! Not in God's eyes. God is sinless. God is Holy. God is pure. He cannot cohabitate with any sin (even as little as you think yours may be).

So how are we ever going to get into heaven if we're so full of sin and God can't be near us? As nurses we can help heal the physical body, but we cannot save the soul. We can help mend wounds, but we can't fix someone's eternity for them so they can live forever without pain and suffering. As much as we may want to, we don't have that ability.

It all sounds hopeless until... Jesus. God loves us enough that He gave the ultimate gift. The ultimate sacrifice was made for you and for me to make us all clean and 100% pure in God's eyes. God sent His one and only son, Jesus Christ, to take on human form (to be fully God and fully human at the same time), die on the cross and take on all of your sin. All of my sin. Everyone's sin, no matter how big or small. He paid the price. You're free. You are forgiven. You are able to spend eternity with God the Father in heaven - the place that is so beautiful and amazing that we cannot even fathom its glory.

1 Corinthians 2:9 says "Eye has not seen, nor ear heard, nor have entered into the heart of man the things

which God has prepared for those who love Him". It's more than we can even imagine.... for those who love Him. That's it. The one and only catch. The one and only thing He asks. Jesus wants you to love and accept Him. That's it. He wants you to believe He is the one true son of God and that He died to pay your debt for sin so you can enter that beautiful eternity free of charge. When we see patients who live with this hope finally take their last breath, it is amazing to think, at that very moment, they are quite possibly entering that place that is more beautiful than we can ever imagine. That's a lot to take in. And just the same, it hurts and saddens me to think of the others who are lost, hopeless and full of despair at the end of their days. That seems so empty, sad and wrong.

> "Greater love has no one than this, than to lay down one's life for his friends."
> -John 15:13

"Greater love has no one than this, than to lay down one's life for his friends" John 15:13. Is there any greater love? Than to give one's own life for another? People praise veterans all the time for this very act (and rightly so!), yet those same people don't always spend much time thinking about what Jesus took for them. Veterans gave their lives to give freedom to you and I in this life. Jesus gave His life to give freedom for all of eternity. He had you and me in mind while He was on that cross. He knows each one of us better than we know ourselves, and His love is more than we can fathom.

The beautiful thing here is that God loves us enough that He does not force this on any of us. He gives us the choice, fair and simple. He did what was necessary to save us, and now we have free will to decide if we want to accept His gift, or not. God doesn't just "make" everyone perfect and force everyone to love Him. He gives us that choice. What kind of relationship would you rather? One where your spouse is FORCED to love you, or one where they choose to love you on their own free will? It seems like the latter is a much more meaningful relationship, don't you think? God deserves and wants the same from us. However, there are many people out there who still choose to reject Him. In doing this, there is much sin and destruction in this life, and many will not make it into that beautiful eternity. God isn't controlling everyone's every move. He gives everyone that choice, including you.

What do you have to lose? Do you have a better plan? Where do you find YOUR hope, if not in Jesus Christ who promises the gift of eternal life? What does your hope promise to you that is greater than the forgiveness of all your sin and the promise of eternity in heaven? I offer this as something for you to think about if you have never done so before.

Not only did Jesus suffer and die on our part, but he beat death itself. He beat DEATH. Jesus was tortured, beaten and hung on the cross to die, and three days later he rose from the dead. Death could not stop Him. This is the power of God. This is the hope we have in Jesus Christ that he has beaten death itself. He has given us victory over sin and death. This is why Easter is so amazing. Romans 6:9 "knowing that Christ, having been raised from the dead, dies no more. Death no longer has dominion over Him". I can't think of anything more powerful than that.

Joy and Suffering

How is it that some people can have such joy in times of suffering? Have you ever seen this with any of your patients suffering with a horrible disease? I have, and it is amazing. You see some of these people going through such awful circumstances and you just can't believe how they are smiling. How do they have peace with all that going on?

What is true joy? Joy is not the absence of your problems, but rather the presence of Jesus in the middle of them. Jesus offers pure joy in our hearts when we accept Him. This does NOT mean your life will automatically become perfect and all your problems will disappear. No. Life is still hard, problems will still happen, and it doesn't mean everything is rosy all the time. But God offers us a peace that passes all understanding. We can't even make sense of it, but it's there, and it's so strong. There is suffering in this world. But when we have the hope of Jesus in our hearts, we can have joy in the midst of our chaos.

This was never made so tangible to me as it was when I went to Kenya. We saw those little children who had absolutely nothing. They wore rags for clothes, had minimal food to eat, and absolutely none of the comforts we enjoy here in our everyday lives. But do you know what they had ten times over most kids I see every day? Joy. Pure joy. Those children danced for joy and sang praises to God. HE was their joy, and that beats having "stuff" any day. That beats having the perfect life you and I think we need by the world's standards. Those kids taught me a huge lesson, and for that I am grateful.

Life is still hard and we all have bad times. But I will say, there is meaning in our struggles and trials even though we may not see it at the time. God uses certain times in our lives to mold us, test us, and shape us into more of who He wants us to be. James 1:2-4 says "My brethren, count it all joy when you fall into various trials, knowing that the testing of your faith produces patience. But let patience have its perfect work, that you may be perfect and complete, lacking nothing". You could be struggling right now. I cannot tell you why, but please don't let your circumstances dictate your belief in God. You may possibly be going through something hard so you are better equipped to help someone else in the future with a similar struggle. What a blessing you could be to someone else, only because you have been refined by your own struggles. Or you may have been badly hurt by a church in your past. Churches are full of imperfect people... we're all a work in progress. Don't let an imperfect human's actions decide your relationship with God Himself who IS perfect.

Temporary vs. Eternal

What are you taking with you when you go? Your body? Nope. Your money? Nope. Your house, car, or dearest possessions? Nope. None of it. Our bodies are temporary, but the Word of the Lord is eternal. Isaiah 40:6,8 says "All flesh is as grass, and all its loveliness is like the flower of the field. The grass withers, the flower fades, but the word of our God stands forever". Our bodies will fail, our "loveliness" will fade, and our possessions will not last forever. Yet so many of us focus all our time, effort and attention on these temporary things rather than what is eternal.

What things do you value here on earth? Show me how you spend your time and money and I will show you where your values are. Are we more interested in getting more "stuff" that we can't take with us anyway? Do we spend our time doing things that have meaning and make a difference in the lives of those around us, or is it all just superficial nonsense that has no lasting value? Putting your time and money into things that have lasting value and meaning can give such a deeper satisfaction than the alternative.

Although your body may be temporary, I would say that's one of the best investments you can spend your time and money on because it needs to last while you're here! Don't skimp when it comes to spending on your own health. Pass on some of the "stuff" and invest in your health and your eternity.

Be Strong

What about strength? I love being strong in a physical sense, but that will only get me so far. Relying on strength from God Himself is a power so far beyond what we can do ourselves. Philippians 4:13 says "I can do all things through Christ who strengthens me". All things. When we reach out for the power of Christ to sustain us, we are able to get through so much more than we ever would on our own. I love seeing patients I have encountered doing just that. Relying on our own strength can only do so much. After all, as we already know, our bodies will fail us at some point. Psalm 73:26 says "My flesh and my heart fail; but God is the strength of my heart and my portion forever".

There are so many amazing scriptures about strength in the Bible. Isaiah 40:29-31 says "He gives power to the weak, and to those who have no might He increases strength. Even the youths shall faint and be weary, and the young men shall utterly fall, but those who wait on the Lord shall renew their strength; they shall mount up with wings like eagles, they shall run and not be weary, they shall walk and not faint". He gives us strength that we could never have on our own. His strength is made perfect in our weakness. Jesus wants to walk right alongside of us in our weakness and He gives us the strength to go on.

Is anyone out there a Rich Froning fan? For those of you not familiar with who he is, Rich Froning has been named the Fittest Man on Earth after winning four back-to-back individual Crossfit Games championships from 2011-2014. Talk about discipline and dedication to fitness, this guy is amazing. Have you ever noticed what he has tattooed on his side? He has the reference Galatians 6:14, which says "But God forbid that I should boast except in the cross of our Lord Jesus Christ..." He is giving all the glory to God, and not boasting of himself. Someone like that could very easily boast of his own strength, yet he outwardly gives the glory to God. I think that's pretty cool.

Staying strong on our own can be hard. Jesus says in Matthew 11:28 "Come to Me all you who labor and are heavy laden, and I will give you rest". Don't we feel like that often as nurses? Don't we feel like that often just in our own lives? We're tired of trying to do it all on our own. We're tired of always trying to live up to the world's standards. We need rest. Jesus offers us that rest. He offers us hope, comfort, and a beautiful eternity with Him. Don't pass that up. If any of this makes you wonder, keep searching it out. Keep asking and seeking. Don't ignore it. You can have that peace, in this life and for eternity.

> **"Come to Me all you who labor and are heavy laden, and I will give you rest."**
> **-Matthew 11:28**

In this day and age with a mobile app for absolutely everything, of course there is a Bible app you can use on your phone or other mobile device. The YouVersion Bible app is a great tool with many reading plans, videos and other helpful ways to get your questions answered, learn more, and grow in this area. Just something to consider if you want or need direction with this.

The new and Improved Nurse

Is it possible to really live better than you have been up until now? I know all that information may have been a lot for some of you to take in all at once. I certainly hope that you can at least take some of what you have read in this book and apply it to your everyday life, as a nurse, and as a great human being. Life is too short to waste time being tired, sick, worn out and hopeless. There is so much more! It's time to feel better and live better. Nurses work too hard to get nothing back in return.

Regret is something none of us want. Please don't get to the end of your life and wish you had done it all differently. You can start today. By taking tips from this book, you can start eating better, move a little every day, get stronger, decrease your stress on the job and at home, avoid toxins in your food and environment, increase your energy, decrease your risk of disease, learn to listen to your body, realize your worth, squash doubt, reach to find your limits, and seal your eternity in a beautiful place called heaven. Wow. That might even sound too good to be true... but it's not! It is truly possible, although it is your choice to take the first steps. No one else can do that for you. But I promise, I've got your back when you make that decision to start!

Start small and make little changes where you can. And by all means, allow for some grace when you mess up. Aim for progress, not perfection. Any forward progress, no matter how small, is still progress! Don't forget that. Perfection isn't necessary, nor is it attainable, so don't waste your time aiming for it.

It's time to take care of the nurse. Become a better version of you. The BEST version of you. Why not? You are important, necessary, and needed in this life. Make it the very best you can. There is a person behind that nursing career that desperately needs permission to be cared for. Learn to love yourself, care for yourself, and yes, even put yourself first sometimes! Invest in your health here on this earth, and by all means your eternity as well. Take care of the "whole self". Mind, body and spirit.

Writing this book has been a passion of mine that has proven to be stronger than I realized. I truly pray for each and every one reading this book. I honestly mean that. If I was able to shed some light, provide encouragement, and motivate any of you in a positive way, then this was all worth it. Live well, be well, and become a Nurse Gone Strong! You got this... God bless!

References

1. American Council on Exercise; *Personal Trainer Manual, Fifth Edition*. California: American Council on Exercise, 2014

2. Borynsenko, J.; *The Plant Plus Diet Solution*. New York: Hay House, Inc., 2012

3. Davis, W.; *Wheat Belly.* New York: Rodale, Inc., 2011

4. Hyman, M.; "5 Reasons High Fructose Corn Syrup Will Kill You", www.drhyman.com/blog/2011/05/13/5-reasons-high-fructose-corn-syrup-will-kill-you/

5. Kresser, C.; "Fifty Shades of Gluten Intolerance", 4/02/2013. www.huffingtonpost.com/chris-kresser/gluten-intolerance_b_2964812

6. Mercola, J; "7 Worst Ingredients in Food", www.articles.mercola.com/sites/articles/archive/2013/12/30/worst-food-ingredients.aspx

7. Minger, D.; "The Truth About Ancel Keys: We've All Got it Wrong", www.denisminger.com/2011/12/22/the-truth-about-ancel-keys-weve-all-got-it-wrong/

8. Reader's Digest; *Fight Back With Food.* New York: The Reader's Digest Association, 2002

9. Sisson, M.; *The Primal Blueprint*. California: Primal Nutrition, Inc., 2012

10. Taubes, G.; *Why We Get Fat and What to Do About it.* New York: Anchor Books, Random House, 2011

Made in the USA
Middletown, DE
11 September 2018